Anna Martha Fullerton

Nursing in Abdominal Surgery and Diseases of Women

Anna Martha Fullerton

Nursing in Abdominal Surgery and Diseases of Women

ISBN/EAN: 9783742812551

Manufactured in Europe, USA, Canada, Australia, Japa

Cover: Foto ©Lupo / pixelio.de

Manufactured and distributed by brebook publishing software
(www.brebook.com)

Anna Martha Fullerton

Nursing in Abdominal Surgery and Diseases of Women

NURSING IN

ABDOMINAL SURGERY

AND

DISEASES OF WOMEN.

A SERIES OF LECTURES DELIVERED TO THE PUPILS OF THE
TRAINING SCHOOL FOR NURSES CONNECTED WITH
THE WOMAN'S HOSPITAL OF PHILADELPHIA,
COMPRISING THEIR REGULAR COURSE OF
INSTRUCTION ON SUCH TOPICS.

BY

ANNA M. FULLERTON, M.D.,

PHYSICIAN-IN-CHARGE OF AND OBSTETRICIAN AND GYNÆCOLOGIST TO THE
WOMAN'S HOSPITAL OF PHILADELPHIA, ETC.

ILLUSTRATED.

PHILADELPHIA:

P. BLAKISTON, SON & CO.

1012 WALNUT STREET.

1891.

PRESS OF WM. F. FELL & CO.,
1220-24 SANSOM STREET,
PHILADELPHIA.

PREFACE.

Many books have been written within recent years on the subject of abdominal and gynæcological surgery, for the instruction and guidance of the medical student and practitioner, yet none but the most meager details—found chiefly in books on general nursing—have been supplied for the aid of the nurse.

The stringent requirements of aseptic and antiseptic surgery demand that nurses and assistants shall coöperate with the surgeon in enabling him to attain the results desired in operative work. Hence a thorough knowledge of the methods by which the best results are to be obtained is essential. At the request of my pupils—and with the hope of meeting this need in other institutions—I have prepared these lectures for publication. The methods recommended are those which have proved useful and successful in the surgical work of the wards of our Hospital. An effort has been made, however, by careful observation of the work in prominent hospitals both in this country and Europe, as also by a thorough study and comparison of the methods advocated by standard writers, to represent the various plans of management which tend to serve the same end.

The chapter on diet for the sick has kindly been prepared by our matron, Miss Sara H. Janvier, and contains recipes for invalid cookery which are taught our nurses in the diet kitchen connected with the Hospital, in which each nurse has a term of service.

I am indebted to Dr. Anna E. Broomall for many practical points in connection with the methods of management set forth in this book; also, to Dr. Susan Hayhurst, Dr. Frieda E. Lippert, and Miss Alice Littell for aid in its compilation. To all who have helped me by friendly counsel and assistance I would express my sincere thanks.

ANNA M. FULLERTON.

Woman's Hospital of Philadelphia,
October, 1891.

CONTENTS.

CHAPTER XI.

CHAPTER XII.

CHAPTER XIII.

CHAPTER XIV.

CHAPTER XV.

CHAPTER XVI.

CHAPTER XVII.

CHAPTER XVIII.

CHAPTER XIX.

CHAPTER XX.

CHAPTER XXI.

ILLUSTRATIONS.

xi

"So kind, so duteous, diligent,
So tender over (her) occasions, true,
So feat, so nurse-like!"

SHAKESPEARE'S CYMBELINE, IV, 5.

"Ask God to give thee skill in comfort's art
That thou mayst consecrated be and set apart
Unto a life of sympathy;
For heavy is the weight of woe in every heart,
And comforters are needed much of Christ-like touch."

UNKNOWN.

NURSING

IN

ABDOMINAL SURGERY

AND

DISEASES OF WOMEN.

CHAPTER I.

THE SURGICAL NURSE.

"A perfect nurse," says the surgeon, J. Grieg Smith, in his celebrated work on Abdominal Surgery, "is a perfect woman, rarely to be had." There are possibilities of perfection, however, in every human being of average health and ability. Both men and women fail oftener in attaining a high degree of excellence in character and work from *indolence* rather than *incompetency*.

"Energy of will—self-originating force—is the soul of every great character. Where it is, there is life; where it is not, there is faintness, helplessness, and despondency." Energy of will is largely a

Qualifica-
tions for
nursing.

matter of self-discipline, and it is one of the first requisites to success in nursing as in other professions.

A serene, sunny disposition is another important qualification in a good nurse, for it serves to produce an atmosphere of quiet content in the sick-room which conduces greatly to the comfort and well-being of the patient, as of all concerned.

Self-forgetfulness, sympathy, cheerfulness, patience, tact, quickness of observation, method and skill in action, implicit obedience and loyalty to her physician—all of which are so essential to the good nurse—are the fruit of long and careful self-discipline combined with practical experience.

Necessity for training.

The surgical nurse should be habituated to the sight of blood. She should be strong-nerved and of steady hand. Sudden emergencies should not throw her off her guard. Thorough training and a knowledge of the conditions which may demand prompt action on her part will enable her to attain the necessary self-possession. Knowledge gives courage. Skill is gained by practice. For the acquirement of knowledge and skill it is essential that the surgical nurse should have a course of training in the wards of a hospital where considerable surgical work is done.

So much does the success of a surgeon's work depend upon the nurse that extreme care should be exercised in the selection of a suitable person to undertake the supervision and after-care of an operative case.

It is to be hoped that the training-schools of our country will greatly increase the number of nurses fitted to assume these important trusts.

Personal cleanliness is essential in every nurse. This does not imply a simple adherence to the ordinary rules for bathing and general care of the person. "Surgical cleanliness aims at the removal of microscopic particles," hence requires a thorough appreciation of the principles of asepsis and antisepsis. The danger of a nurse's carrying disease from one patient to another makes it imperative that her entire body, including her hair, should receive a thorough cleansing between the different cases she may nurse. After the general bath of warm water and soap, the surface of the body should be washed with an antiseptic solution; as, corrosive sublimate (1-1000); Labarraque's solution of chlorinated soda (1 part to 8 of water); or carbolic solution (1–40). The chlorinated soda solution should not be used on the hair because of its bleaching effect. The irritation of the skin produced by any of the antiseptic washes may be prevented by a subsequent plunge or sponge bath of simple warm water.

Surgical cleanliness

The costume of a nurse is another matter of *Costume of nurse.*

great importance. Apart from its being neat and clean, the entire costume should consist of wash materials to insure its being free from contagion. Without previous washing no articles of dress should be worn in attendance upon two different cases.

Disinfection of clothing. Clothing worn at a contagious case should be allowed to soak in an antiseptic solution from one to two hours before its subjection to the ordinary processes of the wash.

Care should be taken to rinse out the antiseptic solutions very thoroughly before boiling the clothing, as the chemical agents ordinarily used might otherwise produce discoloration. Corrosive sublimate (1–1000) and carbolic solution (1–20) are the agents usually employed. A preparation which has been satisfactorily employed in many hospitals for washing infected clothing is the following: Four ounces of sulphate of zinc, and two ounces common salt dissolved in 1 gallon of water. The clothing may be boiled in this for half an hour and lie in the solution from 4 to 5 hours.

The bleaching effect of chlorine prevents the use of this for colored clothing. Boiling the clothing for half an hour would cause its thorough disinfection, but as care should be taken not to subject those who attend to the washing to danger from infection, and since many laundresses cannot be

trusted to boil the clothing, it is a safe plan to subject it to this double process of cleansing. The
methods of disinfection for various articles will be
more thoroughly dwelt upon in another chapter.
I touch upon the matter here in order to impress
the nurse with the fact that a thorough disinfection
of herself is as important as that of her patient and
his surroundings.

During an operation the nurse should wear an Preparation
entirely fresh suit of clothing, and, if she is obliged tion.
to handle sponges or so assist the surgeon as to
come in contact with him or the patient, a large
clean apron and fresh slip-sleeves should be put on
after all things else are in readiness for the operation.
The especial precautions to be taken in the preparation of her hands for her work are as follows :—

The nails should be kept closely cut, the hands Cleansing
and care of
smooth and soft, that they may not feel rough to hands.
the patient as they come in contact with his skin.
Cold cream or a little glycerine rubbed over the
hands at night; or, if the skin be irritated by pure
glycerine, the use of a wash consisting of bay-rum
($\frac{2}{3}$) and glycerine ($\frac{1}{3}$), makes a nice lotion for the
hands.

Work properly done need not spoil the hands,
provided the precaution be taken after washing
them to dry them thoroughly, and to anoint them
as suggested, when rough.

Should the nurse's hands come in contact with foul discharges, a first cleansing with soap and cold water will best help to remove the odor. Warm water with soap may then be used with a nail-brush for more thorough removal of all particles of dirt, and then some antiseptic, as chlorinated soda. In the special cleansing of the hands for surgical work, various methods may be followed. Thus after a thorough cleaning with soap and water for several minutes, the nail-brush being carefully used, the hands may be immersed in an antiseptic wash, which is similarly thoroughly applied by means of a nail-brush around the finger-nails, etc. Pure alcohol may be used, or corrosive sublimate solution 1–1000, or Labarraque's solution 1–8.

A method employed in some hospitals for sterilizing the hands is described as follows: Ten minutes are spent in washing the hands, finger-nails, and fore-arms with brown (oleine) soap and warm water and a moderately stiff scrubbing brush. After washing thoroughly in water and soap, the hands are next immersed in a saturated solution of permanganate of potash, and held there until they are uniformly deeply stained; from this they are transferred to a saturated solution of oxalic acid, which removes the stain in one minute. They are then dipped in plain water and finally laid in a bath

of bi-chloride of mercury (1–1000) for a full minute.*

A nurse should keep her breath sweet. The Care of breath.
existence of a bad catarrh will incapacitate her
for surgical nursing. The mouth and teeth and
the digestive organs should also receive the attention they demand, so that the patient may suffer
no annoyance from their effect upon the breath.

It should not be necessary to remind a nurse of Personal hygiene.
the importance of attention to her own health. An
earnest purpose to attain the highest success in her
work should lead every nurse to so dispose of her
hours of leisure as to keep herself in the best
working order. " This one thing I do," should be
her motto ; and food and drink, clothing, rest, and
recreation should be so adjusted as to train her for
active duty, and for the strain which must often
come to her in the long vigils of the sick-room,
when every sense should be acute to discover the
slightest change in the sufferer, and every faculty
fully alive to the demands of the moment. Acute
conditions demanding the almost constant presence Sole management
desirable.
of the nurse seldom last longer than a few days,
and a well-trained nurse can ordinarily bear the
strain very well for that length of time. Should the
critical condition be protracted, it may be necessary

---

* Dr. H. Kelly.

to have a division of labor by association with another nurse.

It is so much more satisfactory for one nurse to manage a case throughout, that, unless it is imperative, such an arrangement for sharing work should be avoided. The assistance of some reliable member of the family, at times when the patient is not requiring very especial attention, will often permit a most trying case to be carried through with but one nurse's supervision.

The simplest and most wholesome food and drink, regular out-door exercise, sufficient sleep at a time when sleep is legitimate, good sense in the matter of dress, occasional change of scene and thought in the intervals between cases, will help to keep a nurse in good condition for duty.

"What is there in the world to distinguish virtues from dishonor, or that can make anything rewardable, but the labor and the danger, the pain and the difficulty?"—*Jeremy Taylor.*

CHAPTER II.

THE GERM THEORY OF DISEASE.

In order to thoroughly understand the importance of the minute details to be observed in surgical nursing, it is essential that the nurse should know something of the researches of modern science which have developed what is called the "germ theory of disease."

"Germs" or "bacteria" are forms of life so *Description of "germs."* minute as to be singly invisible to the naked eye. Numerous forms of bacteria have, however, been carefully examined and studied through the microscope, and scientists have thus in recent years learned much of their nature and activities. These researches have proved a most valuable contribution to the science of medicine, for through them *Value of scientific research.* it has been found that many of the most deadly processes of disease are due to the irritating presence of special germs and to the changes which they bring about in the human body.

The causation of disease as induced by these minute organisms, and its prevention by suitable management, are subjects of such great import-

25

ance that scientific workers all over the world are
devoting time to the study of bacteria, with the
hope of eventually exterminating some of the

Diseases
and dis-
eased con-
ditions due
to germs.

present most fatal maladies. Thus consumption,
typhoid fever, cholera, diphtheria, and pneumonia
are due to germs, each disease having its own
specific cause. The same may be said of surgical
diseases,—the complications which may arise in the
healing of wounds ; as, inflammations, abscesses,
erysipelas, and the various forms of blood-poisoning.

Properties
of bacteria.

Bacteria exist almost everywhere. They have
the power of nourishing themselves by using certain
portions of dead organic material, leaving the rest
in such form as to be used by other living things.
They also have the power of moving and of repro-

Conditions
necessary to
development
of germs.

ducing their kind. Warmth, moisture, and a certain
amount of organic matter, are the conditions which
favor their development. Most, but by no means all,
forms of bacteria require air ; some, however, can
develop only in the absence of air.

Rapidity of
increase.

Where the conditions are favorable they may
increase with great rapidity. The process of reproduction is as follows : One of the bacteria grows
a little longer, a constriction forms about the middle
which finally becomes a complete partition, so that

Method of
reproduc-
tion.

two distinct individuals are thus formed. These
similarly divide to produce other bacteria, and their

number thus multiplies. These separate bacteria may fall apart or cling together in chains or in masses. The figures giving us the estimate of the rapidity with which they reproduce themselves, seem almost fabulous. Thus it has been authentically stated that a single germ by this process of growth may in twenty-four hours give rise to more than sixteen and a-half millions.

Bacteria are of various shapes ; the most frequent are the round, oval-shaped, rod-shaped, or spiral-shaped. To give an idea of their size it has been said that of one of the most common forms of bacteria (a little rod), were fifteen hundred of them put end to end, they would scarcely reach across the head of an ordinary pin.

Forms under which bacteria appear.

The different species of bacteria are very numerous. These organisms are to be found wherever any form of life can exist—in water, in the atmosphere, in the soil, in our food and drink, especially that which is uncooked; in all the orifices and canals of our own bodies which communicate with the air, wherever dust can go or collect, there are bacteria of various forms in greater or smaller numbers.

Species.

Substances and localities in which found.

When the bacteria are dry they are said to be inactive, as they are not capable of increasing and multiplying as they do where moisture and the special food they need is present. Of the special

Condition in which inactive.

Species that infect wounds.

forms of bacteria which are apt to infect wounds, it has been found that there are two particular species which give the most trouble in the majority of cases. These are round in shape and are called "micrococci." One species in growing forms chains and is called Streptococcus, the other forms clusters like bunches of grapes and is called Staphylococcus.

Streptococcus.

Staphylococcus.

Both these forms of bacteria exist very abundantly in dirty places, even where healthy people live, but especially where the sick are crowded together. Therefore they are especially to be guarded against in hospitals.

Method of infection.

They are found floating in the air or resting with the dust upon any surface exposed to the air. When dust falls upon the open surface of a wound, or any object upon which bacteria rest comes in contact with such a surface, these living organisms lodge in the wound, and if not destroyed grow there, forming poisonous materials called "ptomaïnes," which interfere with the proper healing of the wound. Poisonous materials may even thus gain access to the blood and be carried to distant parts of the body, where they continue to develop. The whole system may then become infected with the poison, causing serious and often fatal results.

"Ptomaïnes."

Pyogenic bacteria.

In the occurrence of inflammatory complications in the healing of wounds, pus in greater or less quantity is apt to be produced. For this reason the bacteria causing such complications are called *pus-forming* or *pyogenic* bacteria.

This representation of the irritating nature of bacteria under especial conditions is not intended to convey the idea that they are entirely destructive in their tendency. Like all things else in nature, they have a special purpose to serve. They break or tear up worn-out material and thus get it in readiness for new uses—much as a pair of scissors will rip up an old garment and get it in readiness for re-fashioning. Only the bacteria, unlike the scissors, accomplish this work of separating the particles of matter by appropriating to themselves certain substances which serve for their own nutrition. *Uses of bacteria in nature.*

It is only when the condition of the body, or any part of the body, is such as to favor the rapid multiplication of these germs that diseased conditions may be induced.

If the standard of health is maintained by due attention to physiological and sanitary principles, even those liable by heredity to special forms of disease may do much to resist the deleterious effects induced by the presence of germs. *Security against their destructive effect.*

We would, therefore, in this connection remind the nurse of the subtle influences of sunlight, fresh air, good food, cleanliness, and cheerfulness, which will enable her, in the care of the severest cases of illness, to successfully meet and resist the attacks of the unseen but ubiquitous foe. *Hygienic precautions.*

CHAPTER III.

ASEPSIS AND ANTISEPSIS.

Definitions of terms. The word " clean " is derived from an old Saxon term, " claene," which signifies " to open, to remove, to separate." The term " cleanliness," therefore, implies a condition of absolute freedom from all extraneous or foreign matter.

Surgical cleanliness refers more particularly to the absence of all germs of putrefactive change.

The words " aseptic " and " antiseptic," so constantly used by the surgeons of the day, come from a Greek root, the word " septos," meaning " putrid." *Asepsis* means literally " without putrefaction." The germs of putrefactive change may never have been present, or if once present, should have been entirely destroyed in any object which is termed " aseptic."

Antisepsis means " against sepsis or putrefaction," and comprises the means or methods by which objects may be rendered " aseptic." Any substance in which all germs have been destroyed by antiseptic measures, is said to be *"sterilized,"* because the germs have been rendered incapable of doing

30

further injury by continued reproduction. The application of a high degree of heat—dry or ·moist —and the use of certain chemical agents constitute the measures by which germs may be rendered harmless.

In sterilizing inanimate things heat is generally employed. Instruments, towels, clothing, etc., may thus be sterilized by either dry or moist heat. In the use of dry heat it is essential to attain a temperature considerably above the boiling point of water,—at least 230° Fahr. (110° C.). In the disinfection of articles supposed to contain spores (the seeds or eggs of bacteria) it is well to employ this degree of heat for 2 hours. Furnaces or ovens of special design are employed for sterilization by this means, as also for the use of steam under pressure. In the latter case the temperature should be raised to 221° Fahr. (105° C.). For office or hospital work instruments must be kept constantly ready for use, and a small sheet-iron oven, heated by gas, such as is used for bacteriological work, may be employed. This is provided with a thermometer and with a thermostat, by which the flow of gas is automatically controlled, so that the heat is maintained within known limits. The instruments should be subjected to this heat for about one hour. With steam, which is more pene-trating than dry heat, ten to fifteen minutes is

Sterilization of instruments, towels, etc

Steam sterilization.

Office oven.

sufficient for purposes of sterilization. It is not uncommon, however, for greater security, to leave the articles in the steamer longer, as for an hour.

FIG. 1.

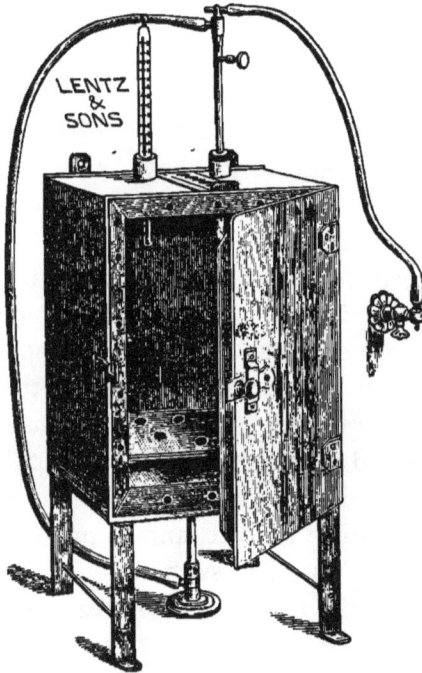

Sterilizing Oven.

Boiling in water for the same length of time is also sufficient, unless the article be bulky, when it is well to extend the time to a half hour. The

Arnold steam sterilizer is perhaps the most con- Arnold steam sterilizer. venient arrangement for the sterilization of instru- ments, towels, etc., and is in use now in most hospitals. It consists of a pan, which contains the water to be heated, communicating with a closed chamber in which the steam accumulates. The articles to be sterilized are placed in this chamber. A double lid is arranged for the prevention of escape of steam. (See Fig. 9.)

Water itself is rendered aseptic by filtering and Sterilization of water. boiling, or distilling and boiling. Distilled water should be entirely aseptic, but its manufacturers rarely appreciate the minute details of asepsis suf- ficiently to take proper precautions to prevent con- tamination. Hence, even when distilled water is employed for an operation, it is well for the nurse to take the precaution of boiling it in vessels which she knows to be clean. Water thus sterilized is made fit for contact with open wounds. Neither rain water nor melted ice will serve as a substitute for water thus prepared, as they are not free from germs.

In the many cases in which heat cannot be used, as in the sterilization of living tissues, chemical agents are employed in solutions of suitable strength, or in the form of powder. The agents thus used are termed " antiseptics," and may be employed accord- Antiseptics.

3

ing to their properties and the strength of their solutions, for one of two purposes,—either as "germicides," true germ-killers, or as "inhibitory agents," that is as substances which check the activity of germs and thus prevent their injurious action. True germicides are so poisonous that they cannot be used except in very dilute solutions when brought in contact with living tissues. In fact, even dilute solutions have been known to cause poisoning by absorption ; hence more and

Asepsis in deep-wound surgery. more in wound surgery the use of boiled distilled water, or boiled filtered water, is replacing the use of antiseptic solutions. Especially is this the case in the surgery of the internal organs. The use of antiseptic washes is more frequent in the

Antisepsis in surface wounds. treatment of surface wounds, accompanied by a foul discharge.

Antiseptic agents in sufficient strength to be germicidal are, therefore, only used for the destruc-

Germicides. tion of germs in putrescent substances outside the body. Thus, *typhoid stools, diphtheritic discharges,* etc., should be rendered innocuous by the strongest germicides available. Such use should be kept entirely distinct from their application in wound surgery.

The following list gives those most commonly employed for germicidal effect.

I. Chloride of lime solution, 4 per cent., made by
adding 6 ounces to the gallon of water.

II. Bichloride of mercury (corrosive sublimate)
solution 1–500, that is 15 grains to the pint.

The above are the best chemical solutions to
employ for the disinfection of *spore-containing
material.*

(*a*) Chloride of lime in powder is a good disinfect- Disinfection
ant for sprinkling over masses of organic of waste
organic
material in privy vaults, etc. It has been matter.
estimated that about one pound of chloride
of lime is required for every thirty pounds of
such material. Should corrosive sublimate
be used for the purpose, one pound of the
powder for every five hundred pounds of
fæcal matter will be sufficient.

(*b*) Slaked lime in the proportion of about one per
cent., that is one pound to the hundred of
the material to be treated, has been shown
recently to be an efficient germicide.

(*c*) Copperas (sulphate of iron), or green vitriol, in
the proportion of 1½ pounds to a gallon of
water, is a valuable agent for the arrest of
putrefactive decomposition, being readily
available because of its low price.

These substances are all of great value where it
is impossible to remove filth from the vicinity of

houses, but they are a poor substitute for cleanliness.

Disinfection of sick-room discharges.

For the disinfection of *discharges in the sick-room*, the solutions ordinarily employed are—

I. Corrosive sublimate (1–500), 15 grains to the pint of water.

II. Chloride of lime (4 per cent.), 5 drachms to the pint.

III. Carbolic acid (5 per cent.), about ¾ of an ounce to the pint.

IV. Sulphate of copper (5 per cent.), about ¾ of an ounce to the pint.

Disinfection of under-clothing, bedding, etc.

Underclothing, bedding, etc., if infected, are best destroyed by fire, if of little value.

To disinfect them, we may employ—

(*a*) Boiling for at least a half hour.

(*b*) Boiling for half an hour in a solution of 4 ounces sulphate of zinc, 2 ounces common salt, to 1 gallon of water.

(*c*) Immersion for three or four hours in a solution of corrosive sublimate, 1–1000.

(*d*) Immersion in a 5 per cent. carbolic solution for the same length of time.

To avoid the discoloring effects of these solutions, clothing taken from them should be thoroughly rinsed out in clear water before it is sent to the laundry.

Outer garments, which would be injured by boiling water or a disinfecting solution, may be sterilized—

(*a*) By exposure to dry heat at a temperature of 230° Fahr. (110° C.).

(*b*) By the steaming process in a suitable apparatus.

Mattresses and *blankets* should be disinfected in the same way.   If these means are not available, mattresses may have their covering removed, and washed and boiled separately, the contents being immersed in boiling water for a half hour.

Furniture, floors, wood-work, painted walls, etc. of a room should be washed with either— Disinfection of furniture, etc.

(*a*) Corrosive sublimate solution (1–1000), which is most efficient, or—

(*b*) Carbolic acid solution 2 per cent.

Rooms are generally disinfected by burning sulphur in the proportion of at least 3 pounds for every thousand cubic feet of air space.   To secure any good results close the apartment as closely as possible by stopping up all apertures through which the gas might escape, by means of wet rags which may be stuffed into the cracks around doors, windows, etc.   The sulphur is put into a deep tin pan which is placed upon two bricks, in a tub partly filled with water, in the middle of the room. Disinfection of a room.

A little alcohol may be poured on the sulphur, which is then set on fire, or a few live coals placed in the pan. The fumes should be kept in the apartment from twelve to twenty-four hours, after which doors and windows should be thrown open, and it should be subjected to free ventilation. All surfaces in the room are then washed off with one of the above-mentioned solutions.

Disinfection of the person. For the disinfection of the *surface of the body*, after a thorough wash with soap and warm water, use may be made of—

    I. Absolute alcohol, as in cleansing the hands (too expensive for general use).
    II. Solution of corrosive sublimate, 1–1000.
    III. Solution of chlorinated soda, 1–10.
    IV. Carbolic acid solution, two per cent.
    V. Saturated solution of permanganate of potassium, followed by the saturated solution of oxalic acid. This should be used for the hands alone, according to the method described in the chapter on the Surgical Nurse.

Cleansing of open wounds. *Open wounds* or raw surfaces are cleansed preferably with boiled distilled water. When dirt has entered the wound, or pus has formed, showing the presence of germs, we may use—

I. Solution of corrosive sublimate, 1–4000, 1–5000, etc.
II. Carbolic solution, 2 per cent.
III. Beta-naphthol solution, 1–2500.

A preparation used much of late for pus-secreting cavities and surfaces, is peroxide of hydrogen (hydrogen dioxide), which has no equal either for safety or efficiency. The compound is so unstable that, unless the bottle containing it be kept very firmly and securely corked, in the intervals of its use, it will lose its virtue. It should always be kept in a dark, cool place, and should not be shaken violently.

For *surgical dressings* we do not so much need germicides as inhibitory agents. The various gauzes as ordinarily prepared with bichloride of mercury, boric acid, carbolic acid, eucalyptus, salicylic acid, etc., serve this purpose, as does the use of iodoform, aristol, or boric acid in powder. Surgical dressings.

Bichloride of mercury, or corrosive sublimate gauze, is that most generally preferred. To prepare it the gauze is allowed to soak for an hour in a sud of soft soap to remove all "sizing." It is then wrung out of clear water several times until the soap is well out of it, and is immersed in a solution of corrosive sublimate, 1–100 (75 grains to the pint of water), or a weaker solution, as 1–1000, may be used. It is then dried in an oven. As Preparation of bichloride gauze.

drying the gauze in this way, especially if the temperature of the oven be raised high enough to bake it, has the effect of rendering it non-absorbent, it is desirable either to sprinkle a little glycerine over the layers of gauze before drying, or to put a small quantity in the corrosive sublimate. solution used in its preparation. After this process the gauze should be kept carefully from dust and contamination by contact with unsterilized substances. It may be rolled in an antiseptic towel for this purpose, and kept in a closed box or drawer.

Protection of surgical instruments during operation. After *surgical instruments* have been rendered aseptic by thorough cleansing with soap and water, followed by the process of baking, steaming, or boiling, they may be kept free from contamination during an operation by lying immersed under—

I. Sterilized water.
II. Beta-naphthol solution, 1–2500.
III. Carbolic acid solution, 2 per cent. or 1–40.

The blackening effect of carbolic acid may be prevented by the addition of a little glycerine to the solution.

The use of iodide of mercury as an antiseptic— a substance used in the same manner as corrosive sublimate—need scarcely be mentioned. The solutions are more troublesome to prepare, and no more efficient, hence their use is limited. Various other substances have been used for antiseptic purposes, but those mentioned here are the most frequently and universally employed.

In the preparations of solutions of corrosive sublimate, chlorinated lime, and copperas, it should be remembered that they have an injurious effect upon metal, hence should be mixed in glass, porcelain, or agate vessels. Large quantities of solution of chlorinated lime may be made in a bucket.

These rules concerning the use of antiseptics should be thoroughly understood by every good nurse, for even the surgeons who employ aseptic methods, as a rule, require the use of antiseptics beforehand, to bring about a perfect state of asepsis for the operation, and to enable the aseptic state to be preserved after the operation.

Relation between asepsis and antisepsis.

CHAPTER IV.

ABDOMINAL SECTION.

Definition. The operation of abdominal section consists in the making of an incision through the walls of the abdomen, by which the surgeon is enabled to perform any operation required upon the organs contained in the abdomen or the pelvis.

Abdominal organs. The abdominal organs are :—

The stomach.
The intestines.
The liver and gall-bladder.
The kidneys and ureters.
The spleen.
The pancreas.

Pelvic organs. The pelvic organs are :—

The uterus, or womb.
The Fallopian tubes.
The ovaries.
The bladder.
The rectum.

Causes for abdominal section. All these organs are subject to disease, to injuries the result of accidents, and to the development

42

of new growths termed "tumors." Hence it may
be seen that an abdominal section may be under-

FIG. 2.

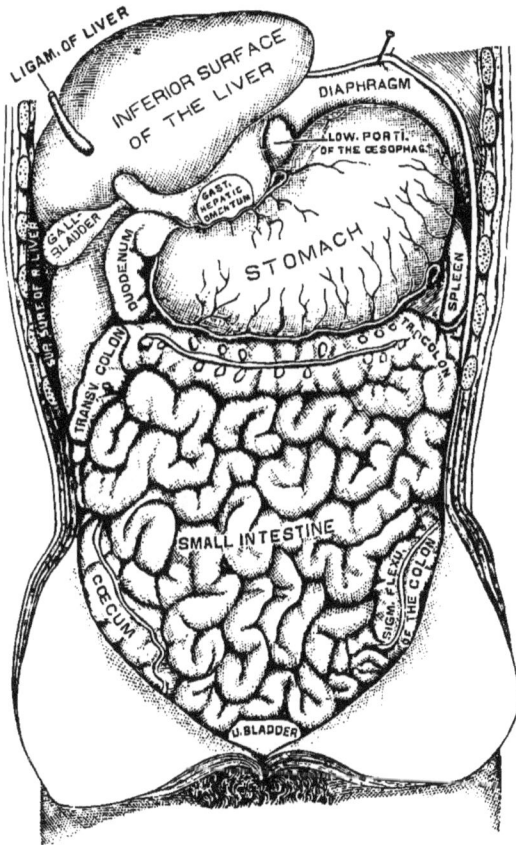

Diagram Showing Abdominal Organs.

taken for very varied conditions. Where no actual disease exists, as in pregnancy, when the birth-track is too small, or there is some other abnormal

FIG. 3.

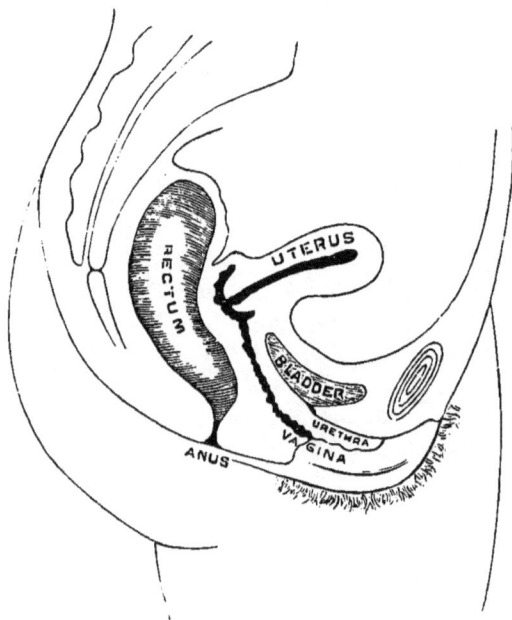

Cut Showing Vertical Section of Pelvic Organs.

condition preventing the occurrence of labor in the natural way, abdominal operation may be per-formed to effect the act of delivery.

The special operation required in each case is known by a distinctive name. Since the nurse's work is closely associated with that of the surgeon, she will constantly hear these terms used. It is desirable that she should understand their meaning .(although it is not necessary, or even in good taste, for her to attempt their use), in order that she may make the necessary preparations in any given case intelligently. For the better understanding of these terms I append a list of the principal abdominal operations :

Operations on the Ovaries and Fallopian Tubes :— Operations on internal genital organs.

  I. Ovariotomy—removal of ovarian tumors.
 II. Oöphorectomy—removal of ovaries of comparatively small size, diseased or healthy.
III. Removal of uterine appendages, when the tubes and ovaries are both removed.

Operations on the Uterus :—

  I. Hysterectomy—removal of the uterus.
 II. Cæsarean section—an incision into the uterus during pregnancy, for extraction of the child.
III. Porro's operation—removal of the uterus, added to Cæsarean section.
IV. Operation for extra-uterine pregnancy, removal of tumor composing the ovum or egg,

when it is found outside of the uterine cavity.

V. Abdominal section for rupture of the uterus.

Operations on the stomach. Operations on the Stomach and Intestines :—

I. Gastrotomy—the making of an incision into the stomach for the removal of foreign bodies.

II. Gastrostomy—the establishing of a tube-like passage into the stomach.

III. Gastrorraphy—the suturing of wounds in the stomach.

IV. Pylorectomy—removal of a part or the whole of the pylorus.

V. Gastro-enterostomy—the formation of a passage between the stomach and duodenum.

Operations on intestines. VI. Duodenostomy—the operation of opening the duodenum, and attaching it to the abdominal wall to form an orifice for the introduction of food.

VII. Jejunostomy—the making of an artificial opening through the abdominal wall into the jejunum, for introduction of food.

VIII. Operation for intestinal obstruction.

IX. Enterotomy—the making of an opening into the intestine.

X. Colotomy—the making of an incision into the colon.

XI. Resection of intestine—the removal of a portion of intestine.

XII. Operation for artificial anus.

Operations on Kidneys :—

    I. Nephrorrhaphy—the suturing of the kidney to the abdominal wall.

    II. Nephro-lithotomy—the operation for removal of stone in the kidney.

    III. Puncture of the kidney.

    IV. Nephrotomy—an operation for opening into the substance of the kidney.

    V. Nephrectomy—removal of the kidney.

Operations on kidneys.

Operations on the Liver and Gall-Bladder :—

    I. Hepatotomy—an operation for opening into the liver.

    II. Cholecystotomy—an operation for opening into the gall-bladder.

    III. Entero - cholecystotomy — an operation in which, after opening into the gall-bladder and intestines, the two wounds are sutured to each other.

    IV. Cholecystectomy—removal of the gall-bladder.

Operations on liver and gall-bladder.

Operations on the Spleen :—

    Splenectomy—removal of the spleen.

Operations on spleen.

Operations on pancreas. Operations on the Pancreas :—

Operation for pancreatic cysts.

Operations on omentum and mesentery. Operations for Tumors of the Omentum.

Operations for Tumors of the Mesentery.

Operations on bladder. Cystotomy, or abdominal lithotomy—an operation for an incision through the abdominal wall into the bladder.

Although the operations mentioned are numerous, the general preparations for any case of abdominal section are so similar that they can be considered under one head. These will include the consideration of the following points :—

I. Preparation of the room.

II. Preparation of sponges, instruments and dressings.

III. Preparation of the patient.

IV. Preparation of the operator and assistants.

V. A nurse's duty during operation.

VI. A nurse's duty after operation and during convalescence.

VII. The management of complications.

CHAPTER V.

THE PREPARATION OF THE ROOM.

In speaking of the importance of obtaining for the patient the best possible surroundings for such an operation a celebrated English surgeon says: " There is no disputing the fact that the best results in abdominal surgery are got in specially prepared rooms or wards. * * * * An ideal room, situated in an open and elevated locality, ventilated with warmed (and perhaps filtered) air, wall and floor impermeable to moisture, and readily and easily washed, and with many other excellences which could be detailed—is rarely in this country at the disposal of surgeons." The operating room.

As a rule, the operation is done in the room which is to be occupied by the patient during the convalescence, unless in a special hospital where the rooms are conveniently arranged with reference to an operating room, and where suitable conveniences exist for transferring patients from one room to another without too great risk.

All the special preparations for aseptic work may be carefully arranged for, yet these cannot secure the results desired, should the operator, assistants, or nurses fail to observe the principles of surgical cleanliness in every detail. On the other hand, with a thorough understanding of these principles, operations of the gravest character may be performed with success in quarters the most unpromising, and in the slums and alleys of a crowded city. Since "necessity knows no law," the surgical nurse must be prepared to convert even the filthy apartment of a tenement house into an aseptic operating room. To this end certain instructions regarding the preparation of the room should be observed.

Dr. J. Grieg Smith tells us, "A well kept bedroom in a home of gentle folks will require nothing changed or removed." Should the surgeon in charge of a case assume the responsibility of this arrangement, the nurse will, of course, observe his Cleansing of wishes in the matter. Should the preparation of room. the room be left to her discretion, she should regard everything in the room with suspicion until she has placed it beyond suspicion in the matter of cleanliness. The room should, if possible, be large and bright, facing the south, and one which can be kept well ventilated and yet comfortably warmed. There should be no stationary wash-stand in the room. If impossible to obtain a room without, the basin should have all its outlets plugged, and be kept filled with some antiseptic solution.

Carpets, curtains, upholstered furniture, every- *Removal of superfluous furniture.* thing that may harbor dust and filth, ought to be removed. If there is any possibility of the existence of infectious or contagious germs in the room it should be subjected to thorough disinfection with the fumes of sulphur. Before the fumes are started the metal fixtures in the room should be well greased with cosmoline, to prevent the injurious action of sulphur upon them. After this the room should be well ventilated. Should an open fireplace or a stove be in the room, keeping the windows open for twenty-four hours or so, while a large fire is kept burning in the grate, will freshen and purify it.

Regarding the use of the spray in purifying the *Use of spray.* atmosphere we quote from Dr. Smith : * "Some surgeons seek to improve the purity of the atmosphere in which the operation is to be performed by making a steam antiseptic spray play in the room for a few hours. There is no strong objection to this; if it does nothing else it lays the dust. But if the room has been properly cleaned and ventilated, and the surrounding air is of the moderate purity and freshness that may be found almost anywhere in England, the spray in the room is perhaps uncalled for. If any objection could be

---

* "Abdominal Surgery."

raised to the proceeding I think it ought to be on the ground of saturating the atmosphere with moisture. Respiration is not so easy in an atmosphere laden with moisture as in one that is dry, and if a patient has to undergo a prolonged and dangerous operation, we should desire to have the recovery from shock promoted by every possible surrounding benefit, one of which is certainly not a wet, depressing atmosphere to breathe."

Should a surgeon desire this procedure carried out, it may be done as follows: A shallow basin filled with the antiseptic solution required may be placed over a gas stove, the steam from which will rise and fill the room. Doors and windows should be kept closed during the process of spraying until the whole apartment has been thoroughly filled with the steam. A special apparatus known as a " steam atomizer " is sometimes employed, and is essential where during the operation it is desired to have the spray directed over the wound. The nurse will need to keep the boiler filled about two-thirds full of water, to renew the antiseptic solution in the bottle from time to time, and to keep the alcohol lamp in good working order.

Sterilization of walls, floor, etc. The walls, as well as the floor, should be well swept, and all pictures removed. If painted it is well to wash the walls with a corrosive sublimate solution (1–1000) or 2 per cent. carbolic acid.

The floor should be washed up with this solution
after it has been well scrubbed.   But little furniture
should be permitted to remain in the room, but this,
with the frames of windows, doors, etc., must be
similarly washed off with an antiseptic solution.
Shades must be taken down, dusted and then wiped

FIG. 4.

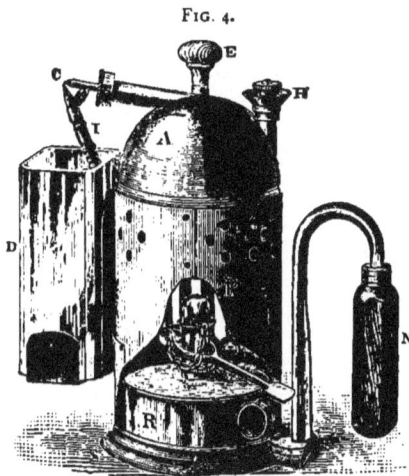

Steam Atomizer.

off also with this solution.   Strips of linen may be
placed on the floor to deaden the footfalls.

The furniture should be conveniently arranged. Arrange-
The bed should be so placed that access may be ment of
furniture.
had to it upon three sides, for convenience in lifting
the patient, changing bedding, etc.   Also, it should

be so placed that the patient shall not face the light from the windows. It should be a single bed, preferably iron, and not too low, with a spring or woven-wire bottom, and a good horse-hair mattress. It is well, if possible, to have two beds, the patient being lifted from one bed to the other, every night and morning, and the bedding thus kept aired. This is not a necessity but a great comfort to the patient. A chair for the nurse and one for the doctor—not rockers—one or two stands, a wash-stand with china set, a bureau with a set of drawers, and one or two large screens, will constitute all that is necessary in the way of furniture. There should be a shade for the lamp, and a quiet-ticking clock placed where the nurse can see it without having to move too much about the room. Inside blinds are the best for tempering the light. There should, if possible, be a closet in the room, in which the various articles needed in the care of the patient may be kept. Changes of clothing, bedding, etc., may be kept in the bureau drawers.

Clothing of patient.   The clothing worn during the operation and subsequent convalescence, should consist of woolen or merino vest, drawers, and socks, varying in thickness with the season, a night-dress of special pattern, extending just below the shoulders in the back, so as to avoid unnecessary and uncomfortable creasing of the clothing, as the patient lies upon her back, the front, pieces should extend down to about the knees. All the articles of dress should be a size larger, or even two sizes larger than those ordinarily worn by the patient, as they are more comfortable to lie in when loose. A Nightingale wrap of light flannel is a convenience for the protection of the shoulders and arms.

The preparation of the clothing, sheets, pillow cases, towels, napkins, etc., previous to operation is as follows : After coming from the laundry, where during the process of cleansing it should have been thoroughly boiled, it is wrung out of a solution of bichloride of mercury 1–1000, or carbolic acid, 2 per cent., when it is dried and smoothed with a warm, not hot, iron, or else left rough dry. Blankets should be either entirely new or they may be hung in a room or large closet, where carbolized steam is generated, as described above. *Steriliza-tion of clothing.*

Three sets of merino wear and night-dresses should be provided to permit the necessary changing of clothing in case of accidents. During the operation it is well to have woolen stockings placed on the patient's feet. These are sometimes worn during the first week or ten days of convalescence.

The bed-clothing is adjusted as follows : Over the mattress is placed a pad for its protection, across the middle of the bed a piece of rubber cloth a yard and a-half wide, pinned down securely to the edges *Arrange-ment of bed-cloth-ing.*

of the mattress. The under sheet or a blanket is then spread over the entire bed, also securely fastened at the corners and edges by safety-pins, to prevent creasing. A draw-sheet (a sheet folded in its length until it is about a yard and a-half in width), is fastened across the middle of the bed, the closed fold of the sheet is directed upward toward the head of the bed to prevent the ridges, which more readily occur when the open end of the sheet is directed upward. The cover-sheet, blanket and spread are then adjusted. Some prefer the patient's lying between blankets for a time; the cover-sheet in such case may be dispensed with.

As the patient may vomit when coming out of anæsthesia it is well to protect the pillow by placing a piece of oil-cloth or rubber around it before drawing on the pillow slip. A towel should be spread over the pillow before the patient is placed in bed, to protect the slip in like manner. If the pillow is not used, as it is often desirable to keep the head low, the towel may be spread over the upper end of the bed where the head will rest.

Muffling of furniture. The stands should have clean cover-slips upon them. The feet of chairs, stands, or any movable furniture in the room should be muffled by twisting with a piece of roller-bandage or soft muslin, so that they may be moved noiselessly; or rubber mufflers may be obtained at large rubber stores for the same purpose. Care should have been exercised beforehand to see that door hinges, latches and window frames, etc., are in proper order, so that there may be no unnecessary rattling or creaking produced by them. It is so essential to keep the patient free from irritation that all these little points should be carefully considered.

A list of the principal articles needed in preparation for the operation will be as follows :— *Articles needed for operation.*

1 strong kitchen table for the patient's body.

1 small table for patient's head.

1 quiet-ticking clock.

Rubber bags for hot water, metal foot-warmers, or soap-stone slabs or bricks for the application of dry heat.

2 basins for catching fluid.

2 large basins or new foot-tubs for sponges.

2 flat trays, metal or hard rubber, for instruments ; basins may be used, though not as convenient.

2 basins for the doctor's hands, to be used interchangeably during operation.

2 waste buckets, large size.

2 buckets cold water.

1 bucket hot water.

1 full wash-stand set.

1 tin cup, graduated if possible.

3 dozen old soft towels.

1 irrigator, either a Davidson hand-syringe, a fountain syringe, or a special contrivance consisting of a funnel, rubber tube, and long hard-rubber nozzle.

1 thermometer for testing heat of water.

1 piece floor oil-cloth for protection of floor.

4 pieces of rubber gum-cloth, 1½ yards square, one for the bed, three for the protection of patient during operation.

1 piece rubber cloth for protection of pillow.

2 pieces of new flannel, ¾ yard wide, 1¼ yards long, for abdominal bandage.

2 pairs woolen hose.

3 sets merino flannels for patient's under-wear.

3 night-dresses.

4 small horse-hair pillows, 8 x 10 in., to use around patient for relief of pressure.

3 new blankets.

½ dozen sheets.

1 spread.

1 or 2 mattresses.

2 pads.

2 large pillows, preferably of hair.

1 pin-cushion with shield and common pins.

1 set of antiseptic dressings.

1 lap absorbent cotton.

1 tray, with tumbler, feeder, teaspoon.

1 medicine glass.

1 clinical thermometer.

1 piece castile soap.

1 new nail brush.

1 vial bichloride tablets for cleansing the hands, etc.

1 pound Calvert's No. 4 carbolic acid.

1 box of matches.

FIG. 5.

Stand for cleansing sponges ◯◯ ◯ Nurse

Stand with Sponges ◯ (Assis. ·tant)

Window

(Chloro. formist)

Table for Patients head

Table for patient's body

Operating Pad

Receptacle for fluid under table extend-ing slightly beyond edge. Flap of opera-ting pad rests over it.

(Operator)

Trays for Instruments

Stand with basin for operator's hands

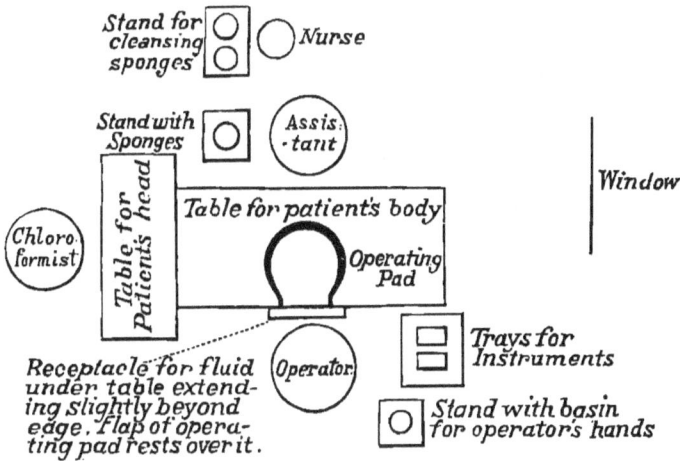

Diagram showing Position, Operator, Assistant, etc., when but one Assistant.

2 or 3 ruled reports.

Pencil and paper for taking directions for after-management.

Arrangement of operating table :—

A table should be placed opposite a window, and

but a few feet from it, unless in a special operating
room where the · lighting of the apartment by
means of a sky-light may enable the table to
occupy the centre of the space.

Various special forms of operating tables have
been devised and are in use in different hospitals.

FIG. 6.

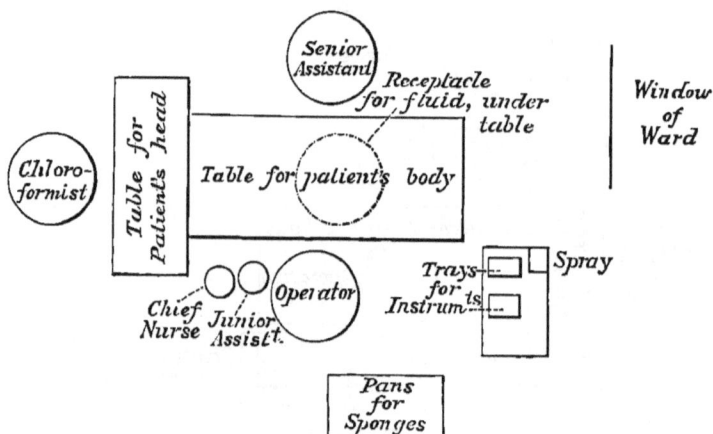

Diagram showing Position, Operator, Assistants, etc., when two
Assistants.

Ordinarily, however, a plain, narrow, wooden table,
such as is used in kitchens in this country, may be
made to serve the purpose very well.   A chair may
be placed at the foot of the table unless the table is
longer than the patient.   This will support her feet.
If it is not high enough, a stool or cushions may
be so adjusted as· to raise the feet and prevent ten-

sion of the abdominal walls. A better arrangement is the use of a small table, placed as in the cut,
for the head.

The table should be covered with a thick, folded
blanket, or comfortable. A large piece of rubber
cloth or table oil-cloth may be fastened across the
middle, or better still, over the entire table, being
fastened to its edges by tacks, to prevent slipping.
In the Woman's Hospital a rubber army blanket
is employed. A sheet is similarly fastened over
this. A pillow protected by rubber is placed at the
head of the table, and a folded blanket and sheet
for covering the patient should be placed at the
foot.

If the carpet has not been removed from the
room some protection must be used under the
table, as a piece of floor oil-cloth, large enough to
extend some distance around the table, or a piece
of drugget or old carpet may be used, provided
they are clean.

In a case of ovariotomy, or any operation where
great quantities of fluid will probably need to be
drawn off, a large foot-tub should be placed beneath the table for the reception of the fluid, also
two basins, to be used interchangeably in receiving
the fluid as it flows from the canula, and emptying
it into the tub.

Since the operator stands on the right side of the

patient, the stand for his instruments should be placed near the foot of the table on the right side. Just back of the operator and a little to the right should be another stand or chair, upon which a basin of water for his hands should be placed, to be used during the operation. The water in this basin should be frequently changed by the nurse, a slop-jar for the soiled water, and a pitcher from which the basin may be replenished may stand beside this table.

The assistant stands opposite the operator, on the left side of the patient; therefore to his right and toward the head of the table should be placed a small stand for holding a basin for the sponges, which, after being cleansed by the nurse, should be thrown into it in warm sterilized water. The nurse's stand with two large basins or small tubs filled, the one with cold, and the other with warm sterilized solution, should be placed a short distance back of this, so that the assistant may readily throw a soiled sponge into the basin containing cold water. The nurse then thoroughly washing out the blood, will rinse the sponge through the warm water, and place it in the basin to the assistant's right. A slop-basin and a tin mug, a pitcher or bucket of warm and one of cold sterilized water should stand by the nurse's table, so that there may be no delay in changing the water.

A basin of water for the cleansing of her own hands should stand conveniently near, either on the stand or a chair, so that in attending to the emptying and re-filling of the basin, she may cleanse her own hands before again touching the sponges.

A small, light basin should be placed under the pillow on the table, to be at hand should the patient vomit. Three or four soft towels to be used by the etherizer may also be placed under the pillow. The irrigator with a pitcher or two of sterilized water of required temperature should be placed to one side, in readiness for use at any time.

The window may be screened by a thin curtain of white muslin or lace fastened across the lower panes, or if necessary to protect the entire window from the intrusive gaze of outsiders, whiting may be painted over the inside of the panes, which will exclude observation, but admit light.

When the operator works with two assistants beside the anæsthetizer the arrangement as indicated in Fig. 6 may be followed.

Immediately before the operation, heated foot-warmers—bricks wrapped with towels or jars filled with hot water—should be placed in the bed, over the site upon which the patient is to lie, and under the covers, so that the bed may be warm for her reception.

A basin containing a block of ice and one or two soft towels may stand near the etherizer, as the application of cold to the head during etherization aids frequently in controlling nausea and diminishing the subsequent headache.

FIG 7.

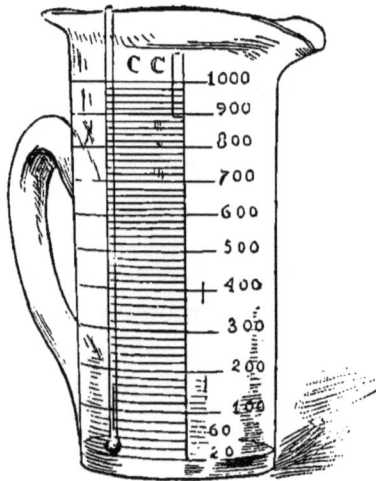

Glass Graduate with Thermometer.

The restoratives which may be needed should the patient sink into collapse should be near at hand—brandy, digitalis, aromatic spirit of ammonia, etc., as the surgeon may desire. A hypodermic syringe in good condition for immediate use should also be provided.

The irrigator or syringe to be used in washing out the abdominal cavity, and sterilized water should be kept in readiness for use when called for. Special receptacles for hot and cold sterilized water may be provided, or a large pitcher full of each, covered with towels to prevent contamination with dust, may be set to one side for the purpose. Another pitcher with distilled water at the required temperature (from 105°–110° Fahr.) should be kept in constant readiness, so that no time may be lost in preparing it.

A bath thermometer, kept in the pitcher, enables the nurse to watch the temperature of the water, and to make an addition to it from time to time from the pitcher of hot water, so as to have it just right when wanted. A large glass graduate with thermometer attachment is used for the purpose in some hospitals.

The Davidson hand-ball syringe used as a siphon will serve as an irrigator where no especial apparatus has been provided. The long rubber vaginal nozzle will need to be used, rather than the shorter nozzles. This syringe and the nozzles should, of course, be perfectly new when used for the purpose.

A representation of a very simple yet efficient irrigator is shown in the cut.

A good plan, where considerable water is likely to be needed for irrigation, is to have three or four

5

pitchers of water of the required temperature ready, so that they can be used in quick succession, or a large glass vessel placed on a shelf, or hung some

FIG. 8.

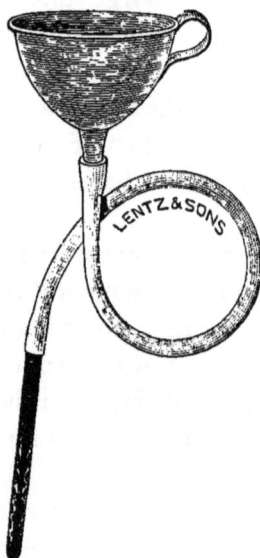

Apparatus for Irrigation of Abdominal Cavity.

distance above the patient, may have the rubber tubing and nozzle attached, and may be kept filled with water of the temperature required.

CHAPTER VI.

PREPARATION OF SPONGES.

The nurse should know something of the nature of sponges, in order to appreciate the necessity for a thorough cleansing of them prior to their application to surgical uses. The sponge is an animal found in the various seas, the fresh water forms being found in rivers and lakes. What we call a sponge is the skeleton of the animal. There are various species of sponges, some being much finer and softer than others. The latter are especially well adapted for use in delicate surgical work. These come to us largely from Turkey and are called the Levant sponge. The Dalmatian sponge is also a fine sponge. A similar species, though not quite so fine, is obtained from the Mediterranean. Two other species, the horse sponge and Zimocca sponge, of coarser quality, are also obtained from the Mediterranean. Florida sponges have of late grown much in favor, and are of a variety of species, some of which are very fine. Sponges grow at varying depths beneath the water, fastening themselves to rocks, stones, and other

Description of sponges.

Whence obtained.

Methods of collecting and preparing for the market. objects. The methods for obtaining them are by harpooning, diving, and dredging. After they are taken from the water they are exposed to the air for some hours until they show a tendency to decomposition. They are then beaten with a thick stick, or trodden by the feet in a stream of flowing water, until the skin and outer soft tissues are completely removed.

After this cleansing they are hung up in the air to dry and then pressed into bales. If the sponges Diseased sponges. are packed before they are thoroughly dry a disease, shown by the presence of orange-yellow spots, breaks out among them. This is called the "sponge cholera," or "pest." Some sponges are naturally of a dark brownish red near the base. This must be distinguished from the disease spots.

In wholesale houses for selling sponges they are cut in shape and further cleaned. The light-colored sponges seen in drug stores have been bleached by the use of chemicals. Sponges are sold by weight, hence sand is often used as an adulteration.

The preparation of sponges in quantity, for hospital use. For hospital use sponges may be bought in 25 lb. bales, bleached and purified. When thus obtained and prepared they probably cost about ¾ cent each when ready for use. For private operations the surgeon usually provides his own sponges and attends to their preparation.

The methods for cleansing sponges, as obtained by the bale, is as follows :—

FOR CLEANING NEW SPONGES.

Method No. 1.—They must first be pounded in an iron mortar, or upon a flat stone, to break up any particles of sand they may hold. Should they be very sandy it is well to soak them in a solution of muriatic acid (2 drachms to the pint) for a few hours. Wring them out in several clean, filtered waters until the water remains perfectly clear. Then immerse in a saturated solution of permanganate of potassium for an hour. After bleaching them with a ten per cent. solution of sulphurous acid (which does its work in an instant), again wring them out in several clean, filtered, and sterilized waters until the water remains perfectly clear and transparent.

Method No. 2.—After ridding the sponges of their sand according to the method described, wring them out of several clean waters. Then immerse in a saturated solution of permanganate of potassium for an hour. Next put them into a saturated solution of oxalic acid and let them remain in this until bleached. They must then be rinsed in several waters (the water being filtered and boiled) until the water is perfectly clear.

Methods for cleaning and rendering aseptic new sponges.

TO CLEANSE OLD SPONGES.

Method for cleansing old sponges. After washing them in cold water to remove the blood, let them soak from 10 to 12 hours in a saturated solution of baking soda, to free them completely of animal matter. Rinse in several waters, and immerse for an hour in the saturated solution of permanganate of potassium. After bleaching them with a saturated solution of oxalic acid, rinse them in several clean waters (boiled and filtered) until the water is clear.

Of the methods described the first produces the prettiest sponges, as the bleaching process is more complete with the sulphurous than with the oxalic acid. Should the sponges during an operation get into a bichloride of mercury solution, it will be found that in recleansing them the sulphurous acid Discoloration of sponges. cannot be used, a chemical reaction causing a darkening of the sponge, so that, although clean, it looks unfit for use.

Storing sponges. After cleaning, sponges may be stored until needed in tightly covered glass jars, being immersed either in alcohol or in a solution of carbolic acid 1–40.

Preparation for operation. Before operation the sponges thus stored should be thoroughly rinsed out in sterilized water and placed in a basin containing warm sterilized water until wanted.

The number of sponges to be used during operation should be carefully counted and recorded on a piece of paper, placed in some conspicuous place for the operator to see. An addition should never be made to the number of sponges in use during an operation without a corresponding change in the number marked on the paper. A sponge should never be cut in two without a similar precaution, as this will change the count, and a sponge may thus be lost sight of and allowed to remain in the abdomen. *Importance of recording numbers used during operation.*

When the operator is ready to close the abdomen all the sponges should be counted by the nurse in a clear, loud tone, so that he may be assured that all are accounted for. *Counting of sponges.*

The assistant, as a rule, takes the sponges out of the warm water and squeezes them dry as he desires them. Should this office devolve upon the nurse, she should see that they are well freed from moisture, and that they are warm when handed to the surgeon.

Sponges which are to be carried down into the abdomen for cleansing it should be mounted on rods called sponge-holders. Three or four of these should be in readiness. They will be needed at the close of the operation and must be handed in rapid succession as wanted. When thus placed in holders or forceps they are called "mounted sponges." *Mounted sponges.*

Flat sponges are used for protecting the intes- *Flat sponges.*

tines, or for application of heat to the abdominal wall. It is well to keep these flat sponges in a separate basin of hot water, handing them when needed. Large squares of flannel wrung out of hot water are sometimes used in place of sponges for application of heat to the abdomen, or for covering over coils of intestine or omentum that may be drawn out of the wound during the course of an operation.

Artificial sponges.

Artificial sponges are made by enclosing balls of sterilized absorbent cotton in sterilized gauze, fastening this firmly with a few stitches so as to perfectly enclose the cotton. These balls may be made of varying sizes. They are used but the once and are thrown away or burned after the operation. They are largely used in place of the natural sponge in many of the hospitals in this country, hence the nurse should learn how to prepare them. She may also thus learn how to improvise sponges for use in a private house, in case of any emergency which may require them.

CHAPTER VII.

STERILIZATION OF INSTRUMENTS, ETC.

The nurse receives the instruments from the surgeon and subjects them to a process of sterilization by wrapping them in a clean dry towel and laying them in a dry or a steam sterilizer, according to the operator's wish.

If dry sterilization is used, the temperature will require to be at least as high as 110° C., or 230 Fahr. Dry sterilization.

In the steam sterilizer a temperature of 100°–105° C., corresponding to 212°–221° Fahr., is sufficient. Steam-sterilization. The rule in most hospitals is to keep the instruments in the sterilizer for about one hour, immediately preceding operation. At the time of the operation the instruments may be lifted out, and the towel around them being loosened they may be allowed to slip into sterilized trays containing warm sterilized water. The nurse's or assistant's hands should be thoroughly disinfected before this is done.

The method of sterilizing the dishes or trays which are to contain the instruments, is as follows : Sterilization of instrument trays.

73

They should first receive a thorough cleansing with soap and warm water, and then should be filled with some strong antiseptic solution, as 1–500 or 1–1000 bichloride of mercury—if of rubber or porcelain; if metal, a solution of carbolic acid 1–20, or of beta-naphthol 1–2500 should be used.

Immersion of instruments in antiseptic solution.

FIG. 9.

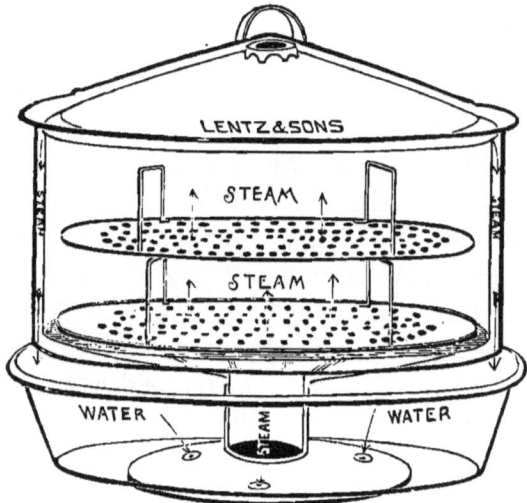

Arnold Steam Sterilizer.

This may stand in the trays until they are needed for the instruments, when the antiseptic solution being emptied out is replaced by boiled distilled, or filtered water. The trays should be about half full, so that the instruments may be well covered.

All the towels and sheets in use around the patient should be sterilized.   Having been carefully
laundried, they should be placed in the steam
sterilizer for an hour preceding the operation, from
which they can be removed as required for the use
of the surgeons.   In some hospitals they are sterilized in quantity and stored in glass jars containing
3 per cent. carbolic solution.

When steam sterilization or dry sterilization
cannot be effected for want of means, the towels,
etc., after a thorough boiling may be soaked in a
solution of bichloride of mercury 1–1000, or
carbolic acid 1–20, and carefully dried in an oven
or clean drying-chamber.   After this they should
be kept free from dust in large glass receptacles or
closed boxes, or they may be stored in a carbolic
acid solution.

The sterilization of cheese-cloth or gauze, and
the preparation of bichloride gauze has already
been given in detail in the chapter on Asepsis and
Antisepsis.   The same formula may be followed
in the preparation of carbolized gauze, borated
gauze, etc.   The strength of the solution of the
special substance to be used in each case will be
given the nurse by the surgeon, should he require
her to prepare the dressings.   As a rule the strength
of the solution used in the preparation of the gauze

is the same as the strongest solution of the agent as employed in irrigation.

Iodoform gauze.

The formula for iodoform gauze is somewhat different. Methods for preparing it vary somewhat, but the following has been found very satisfactory: Six ounces of a 1 per cent. solution of carbolic acid and sterilized water should be prepared, to which is added sufficient castile soap to make a sud. Twelve drachms of iodoform powder should be thoroughly mixed with this. Three yards of gauze previously sterilized by steaming, baking, or boiling, may be prepared by saturating with this mixture. A basin, graduate, and glass rod, which have been previously sterilized, should be used in the making of the mixture and the preparation of the gauze. The same rule should be observed in drying this gauze in the oven as before stated, that is, that a little glycerine should be sprinkled over it to prevent its becoming non-absorbent. The gauze may be cut and preserved in glass jars while moist.

Provision against contamination of antiseptic dressings.

In cutting gauze into strips of the desired length, care should be taken not to contaminate it. A sterilized towel may be spread over a piece of rubber cloth which has previously been cleaned with some antiseptic solution; the gauze may be laid down upon it and cut into the desired strips with a pair of sterilized scissors. The hands of the nurse should be thoroughly disinfected prior to the operation of cutting the gauze. Strips of Sizes of strips. gauze 6 to 8 inches long and 4 inches wide are of good size; also pieces of gauze 4 inches square, some of which are folded so as to make triangles. These are especially nice for tucking around a drainage tube or serre-nœud. A large pad of several folds of gauze, or a pad of sterilized absorbent cotton enclosed in gauze, and large enough to cover the whole abdomen should be in readiness. To prevent handling the dressings, the strips of Storing of antiseptic dressings. antiseptic gauze may be preserved in glass ointment jars of large size with glass lids, such as are used in drug stores. The nurse can then simply remove the lid and hold the jar near the surgeon, enabling him to help himself to the pieces as he needs them.

A many-tailed bandage of new flannel and a pin- Many-tailed bandage. cushion with safety pins will be necessary.

The bandage, with the pad and strips of gauze Special dressings. and a piece of rubber dam about 16 inches square (also sterilized by soaking in carbolic or bichloride solution), with a sponge or sterilized cotton to be placed over the drainage tube, should be wrapped in a sterilized towel and placed to one side until needed, when the nurse should bring them to the operator. If a drying powder, such as boric acid Drying powders. or iodoform, or the two combined, is used it is best kept in a pepper-box or a small box with a piece of gauze tied over the top, so that the powder may be dusted on to the wound.

Method of making many-tailed bandage.
The bandage should consist of a piece of new opera flannel (canton flannel or even thick muslin can be used). This should be properly shrunken. A piece sufficient for one bandage should be about ¾ yard wide and 1¼–1½ yards long. The sides should be torn toward the centre into five strips of equal width. A square of unbleached or any firm muslin, large enough to extend well beyond each side of the patient's loins, as she lies upon the bed, may be used as the base on which the middle portion of each one of five separate strips of flannel may be sewed. The strips should be closely basted on, each overlapping the preceding strip about ⅓ of its width. The muslin may be turned over the edges of the highest and lowest strip. The square of muslin and the strips should be whipped with cotton at the edges and not hemmed, as this makes an uneven surface to lie on. The bandage should be made longer or shorter according to the size of the patient. The object of the muslin square is to prevent the disagreeable sensation of flannel next the skin, particularly as in lying upon it the back is apt to become much heated.

In putting this bandage on, it should be so

arranged that each succeeding strip overlaps the one already adjusted, starting from the upper part of the abdomen. Some surgeons use a perineal pad in addition to the abdominal dressing. In that case a pad of sterilized gauze or cotton may be applied over the vulva and held in place by means of a napkin or towel fastened to the lower border of the abdominal bandage, both anteriorly and posteriorly. *Application of bandage.* *The perineal pad.*

A word or two further may be said in this connection concerning the india rubber cloth used for protection of the drainage tube. A piece about one foot and a half square is necessary. A very small hole is cut in the centre of the cloth. The edge of the hole in the cloth is slipped over the rim of the tube and grips the neck of the tube. If properly put on this rubber cloth will catch any fluid which may escape in such quantity as to soak through the sponge or dressing placed over the mouth of the tube. At each dressing the nurse has simply to turn down the covers of this cloth, which had been folded over the tube and pinned. The tube is thus made accessible. The sponge, when used to cover the orifice of the tube, should be a small conical sponge. During the drainage of the tube this sponge should be kept in an antiseptic solution until it is again needed. *Rubber-dressing.* *Protective sponge.*

In hospital practice particularly it frequently de-

Ligatures and sutures. volves upon the nurse to prepare, or assist in preparing, the ligatures and sutures.

Ligatures are strands of silk or cat-gut, etc., used in tying bleeding vessels, or separating tumors, diseased organs, etc., from the tissues to which they are adherent.

Sutures are strands of various materials, silver wire, iron wire, silk, silk-worm gut, cat-gut, etc., used in approximating the edges of wounds.

Quality of silk. The silk used in abdominal surgery is generally the best quality of " Surgeon's Cable Twist." Three sizes are usually required : fine for the superficial sutures ; medium, or intermediate, for the deep sutures; and heavy for pedicles. This is the best silk for minor operations as well.

Cat-gut. Cat-gut comes in similar sizes, and is required in the three kinds for the same purposes, if the surgeon prefers its use to silk.

These should be wound on separate glass reels for sterilization before use.

Steriliza-tion of silk. The reels containing silk should be put into glass tubes, like test-tubes, containing a wad of cotton in the bottom. The mouth of the tube should be plugged with cotton. The tubes may then be placed in a steam sterilizer or sterilizing oven for a time on three successive days—for one hour the first day ; ½ hour on the second and third days. It is said that thus sterilized it will keep indefinitely.

This method, as well as the following for the preparation of cat-gut, is employed by the surgeons in Johns Hopkins Hospital.

Soak the cat-gut in bichloride of mercury solution 1–1000 for one hour, then in absolute alcohol one hour. Following this, soak for 48 hours in oil of juniper and wind on glass reels. For ½ hour before use the reels of cat-gut may be placed in a jar containing alcohol and boiled in a water-bath. *Preparation of cat-gut.*

Ligatures should be cut both of silk and cat-gut, bunched and wound together, and placed in tubes for sterilization. Care must be taken to observe the different methods in sterilization of silk and cat-gut.

Tubes should be prepared containing only one size of ligatures. When sutures or ligatures are wanted from a tube, the quantity needed may be removed and the tube replugged. The length of ligatures will vary with the requirements. Short ligatures of fine silk or cat-gut, 6-8 inches in length, are used for tying superficial vessels. A medium thickness will be needed for deeper and larger vessels, and the thickest strands for ligating the pedicles of tumors, etc. The latter ligatures will need to be from 40 to 50 inches long, as the pedicle must frequently be divided and the ligatures used to enclose considerable tissue. *Preparation of ligatures.*

Silk-worm gut and silver wire may be cut in

6

Steriliza-
tion of silk-
worm gut
and silver
wire.

proper lengths, 8–10 inches, and bunched together and doubled into test-tubes for sterilization, according to the same process as silk.

" Ignition
tubes."

The glass-tubes used for this purpose, which have recently been devised, have been called "igni-

FIG. 10.

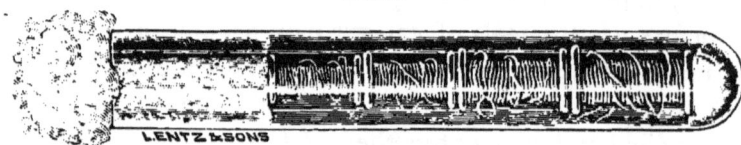

Ignition Tube containing Glass Reels wound with Silk, etc.

tion tubes," and have the advantage over ordinary test-tubes in their greater durability.

Gauze for
capillary
drainage.

Should capillary drainage be employed the nurse will need to prepare pieces of gauze cut into nar-

FIG. 11.

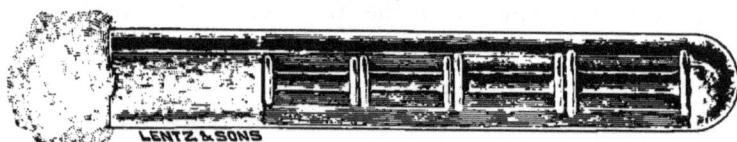

Ignition Tubes for Sterilizing Ligatures, etc., containing Glass Reels.

row strips in suitable lengths for drainage tubes. These should be sterilized in ignition tubes, similarly plugged and used as required in the changing of the dressing.

A sufficient supply of sterilized dressings, gauze, cotton, etc., and another bandage should be kept in readiness for changes subsequent to the operation. These should be carefully guarded from all contamination, hence should be wrapped in a sterilized towel and kept in a closed box or drawer, or, if possible, in closed glass jars.

The threading of needles for the operation sometimes devolves upon the nurse. In that case a tray with the needles already threaded and the ligatures and reels of sutures properly arranged should be in readiness for the surgeon. Long straight glovers' needles are those ordinarily used in abdominal section for the deep stitches. If the surgeon desires, these should be threaded at both ends. Four or five sets of these sutures at least should be prepared, as there is often considerable delay in rethreading. For the superficial stitches a smaller glover's needle with fine suture will be required. Curved needles may be preferred by some operators. The large needles are frequently used without being placed in a needle-holder. The smaller ones the nurse should place in the holder before she hands them to the physician. In seizing the needle in the holder care should be taken not to grasp it directly over the eye, but just beyond it, as the eye is apt to split from the pressure. *Threading of needles.* *Method of seizing needle in holder.*

The silk and cat-gut may be carried through the

eye, and occasionally silk-worm gut and wire are also thus threaded. In the latter case the strand should be carried but a short distance through and bent into a sharp angle at the point where it passes through, so that it may not catch on the tissues in passing through them. Silk-worm gut and wire are usually drawn through the tissues by the aid

Carriers. of strands or loops of fine silk, called "carriers," into which the angle, made in the bent silk-worm gut or wire, may be hooked. The loop is made

FIG. 12.

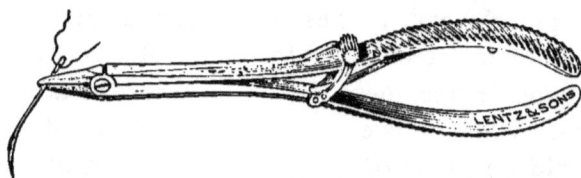

Needle-holder.

by passing the ends of the silk through the eye on the same side of the needle, crossing them and tying around the needle in a small knot.

Pedicle ligatures. Ligatures for the pedicle are threaded into an instrument with an eye at the point, called "a pedicle needle." The operator usually has two or three of these. The long ends of the silk should be twisted around the instrument to prevent tangling, until the ligature is needed.

A list of the instruments most commonly employed for abdominal operations is as follows :—
Scalpel.

FIG. 13.

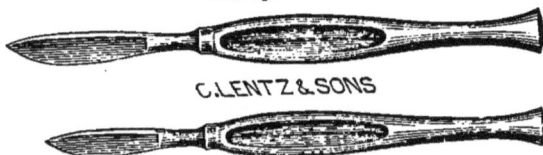

C.LENTZ&SONS

Scalpels.

Knife.
Hæmostatic, or pressure forceps.

FIG. 14.

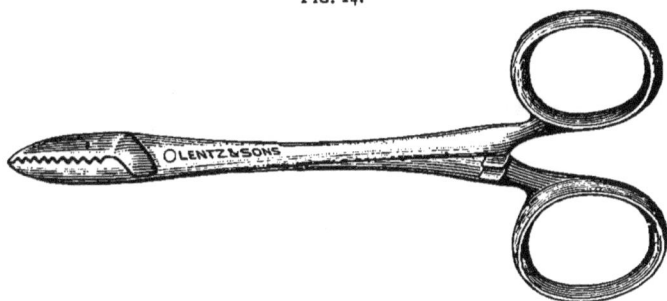

Pressure-forceps.

Grooved director.

FIG. 15.

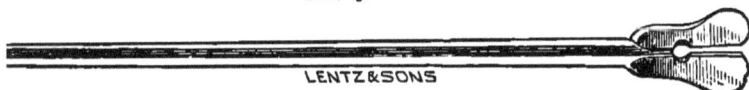

LENTZ&SONS

Grooved Director.

Scissors (curved, straight, or angular).

FIG. 16.

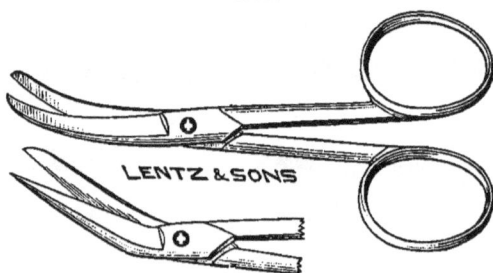

Curved and Bent Scissors.

Trocar.

FIG. 17.

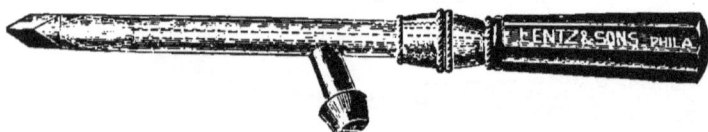

Trocar and Canula.

Volsella.

FIG. 18.

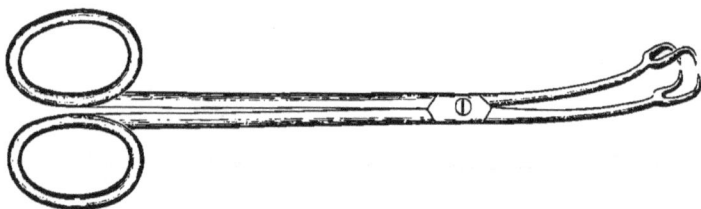

Volsella.

Cyst forceps, or large pressure forceps, straight.

FIG. 19.

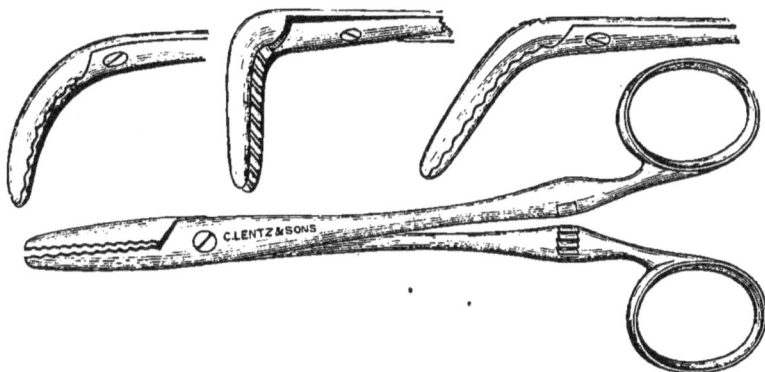

Cyst Forceps.

Bent pressure forceps.
T   "   "

FIG. 20.

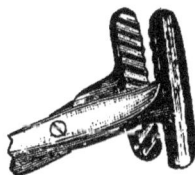

T Forceps.

Retractors.

FIG. 21.

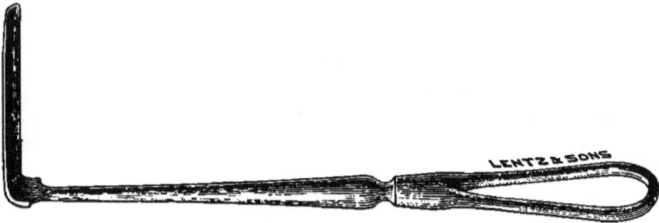

Retractor.

Pedicle needle.

Needle-holder (see Fig. 12).

FIG. 22.

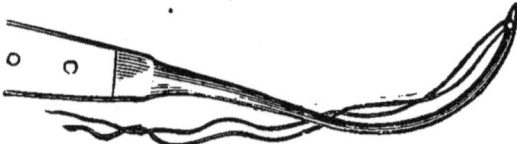

Pedicle Needle.

Serre-nœud.

FIG. 23.

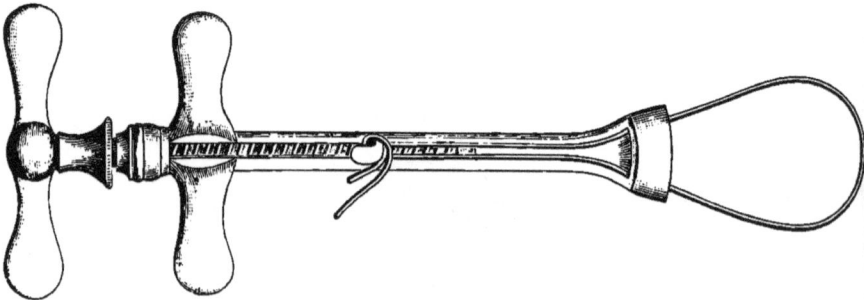

Serre-nœud.

Pedicle pins.

FIG. 24.

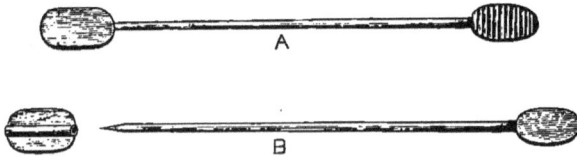

Pedicle Pins.

Drainage tube.
Syringe for draining tube.
Needles.

CHAPTER VIII.

PREPARATION OF THE PATIENT.

Necessity for previous preparation. It is well, if possible, to have the patient under observation some days before operation, in order that she may have a thorough physical examination, and also that the functions of skin, kidneys and bowels may be stimulated to their proper activity, if they have, as is so often the case, been sluggish from improper habits of living.

Daily bath. If the patient is in fair condition a daily warm bath, with a thorough cleansing of the skin with soap and water, will be of advantage. On the day of the operation particular care will have to be taken in the cleansing of the site of the operation. This process will be described later.

Daily vaginal injection. A daily vaginal injection of some antiseptic solution is desirable.

Daily evacuation of bowels. A daily evacuation of the bowels should be obtained by careful regulation of the diet, or, if necessary, by the use of laxatives and enemata as prescribed by the surgeon.

Character of food. The meals should be of such character as to leave as little residual matter in the bowels as possible.

Hence broths, milk, eggs, etc., should constitute a large proportion of the dietary. The patient should be well fed, but a careful selection of the articles for her meals should be made.

The day before the operation it is well to employ a purge—one of the salines is usually employed for the purpose, as a tablespoonful of Rochelle or Epsom salts by mouth; or the surgeon may prefer the use of a saline by enema. *Preparation of bowels immediately before operation.*

A combination frequently used by us is the following :—

2 tablespoonfuls of Rochelle or Epsom salts.
2   "   " Castor oil.
1   "   " Turpentine.
1   "   " Glycerine.
1 pint of water (105° F.).

These should be thoroughly mixed and carefully injected into the bowel. As a rule the bowels act freely within a short time after this injection has been received. To prevent any possible irritation of the bowel a small quantity, as 1 gill of saline solution (½ teaspoonful of salt to 1 gill water), may be injected into the bowel and retained after a free evacuation has been obtained. Should the salts be given by mouth the evening before an operation, a simple enema of soapsuds on the following morning will be sufficient to produce a satisfactory evacuation.

Special preparations on day of operation.   On the morning of the operation a full bath should be given—a plunge bath of soap and warm water, if the patient is strong enough.   If not, a sponge-bath may be given as the patient lies in bed.

The abdomen should be shaved of all hair, particularly the pubes.   It is well to ask the surgeon whether he desires this done or not, as some sur-

FIG. 25.

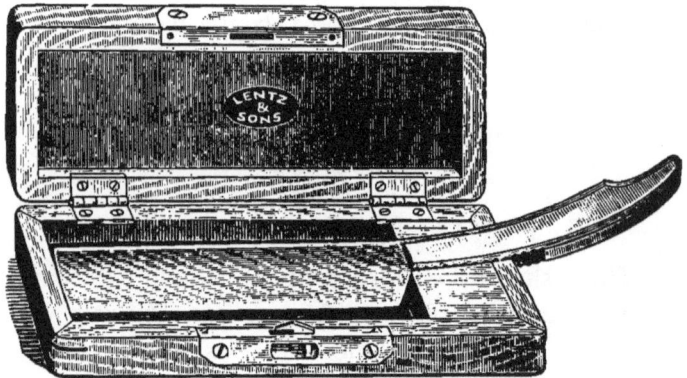

Aseptic Razor with Metal Handle.

geons prefer doing it after etherization, if done at all.

Cleansing of site of operation.   Cleanse the abdomen of all grease by rubbing over it a little turpentine, alcohol, or ether.   This should be followed by again washing with warm water and subsequently with the antiseptic solution 1–1000 bichloride of mercury.   After this a dressing, wet or dry, of some antiseptic gauze should be bandaged over the part and kept in place until it is time for the operation. In this cleansing the umbilicus and pubes should be especially well scrubbed with a nail brush; all particles of dust and dirt should be gotten rid of.

The patient's hair should be arranged in two braids, one immediately behind each ear, the hair being parted all the way down the back. This gives the patient a smooth surface to lie on, and prevents the matting of the hair, which is so apt to occur with any long-continued illness. Arrangement of hair.

Earrings should be removed, as they may catch in the clothing, and, if the patient struggles while taking ether, the ear may be torn. False teeth should be removed, whether whole sets or single teeth, as they may be swallowed during etherization. They should be put away in a safe place. It is best to keep them immersed in a little fresh water. Removal of earrings, false teeth, etc.

The patient should have on an entirely fresh suit of clothing, a merino undervest opened all the way down the front and brought together by tapes fastened two or three inches back from the edges, so that no gap may be left between when the tapes are tied. Merino drawers and woolen stockings should be worn and a night gown of especial pattern, having a short back-piece which reaches just Clothing of patient.

below the shoulders, the front of the gown being long enough to reach to the knees. This avoids the thick folds and creases under the patient's back which the ordinary long night gown is so apt to produce.

At least three suits of clothing should be prepared to have sufficient for the changes that may be necessary. The clothing should be of a size larger or two sizes larger than that ordinarily worn by the patient, as loose clothing is so much more comfortable to lie in.

Evacuation of bladder. The patient should pass water before operation, so that the full bladder shall not be in the way of the operator. If there is some abnormal condition which prevents her passing water, the catheter may have to be passed. But this is best done after etherization, both because it gives the patient less annoyance and because it is desirable to accurately locate the bladder at the time of operation.

Antiseptic vaginal injection. A vaginal injection of bichloride of mercury 1–4000, should be given just before the operation. Occasionally the operator prefers to have it given after the patient is placed upon the operating table.

These preparations should be made in some other than the operating room, and the patient, after she is ready, may lie down on a bed between sterilized sheets until she is etherized.

The patient should take no food on the morning

of the operation. If the operation is not to take place until noon or later, a cup of hot coffee or tea, according to her choice, may be given her. Milk should be avoided because of its tendency to form curds (especially under the effect of strong nervous excitement), which may remain in the stomach, and being vomited during etherization tend to choke the patient. The patient should remain in bed on the morning of the operation, to avoid feeling faint for want of food.

Coverings.—During the operation the patient should be so wrapped that as little as possible of the body heat shall be lost.

A warm blanket may be folded over the lower limbs, or wrapped around them and fastened with safety pins, if it is desired thus to keep the limbs immovable. If the surgeon desires to be able to separate them or bend them from time to time, they may be separately wrapped and pinned in blankets. The clothing of the chest should be folded back, being drawn above the shoulder-blades and on a level with the breasts, and thus fastened with safety pins. The sleeves may similarly be rolled up above the elbows, sterilized towels being twisted around the uncovered portion of the arm, the end of the twist at the wrist being tucked under the patient's body as the arms are stretched out at her sides. A different disposition of the arms will be required if the operating pad is used. They may in the latter case be bent at the elbow, the fore-arms resting upon the pillow and covered by the clothing of the chest. A blanket or a piece of flannel may be placed over the patient's chest, or a layer of cotton wool may be put under the merino vest. If it is necessary to take extra care about keeping the patient warm, a rubber bag filled with hot water may be placed at her feet, or rolls of wool wrapped around the limbs under the blankets.

Protec-
tives.
Different surgeons have various devices for protecting the patient's clothing during operation. Special pads of rubber may be adjusted under the patient's back and thighs, which will serve to carry off the water used in irrigation or any liquid spilled. A very simple and effectual arrangement is that afforded by three sheets of rubber protective, each 1½ yards wide and 2 yards long. One of these may be slipped under the patient's back, covering the arms at the side, the ends hanging down over the sides of the table. Another is so adjusted as to cover the chest, being folded under the clothing front and back.

Towels may be so arranged in covering the rubber that it does not come in direct contact with the skin. The third piece of rubber sheeting covers the blanket over the lower limbs, being turned down over the edge of the blanket on a line with the pubes. A sterilized sheet may be spread over this rubber sheet and similarly turned down. Sterilized towels may then be placed on the chest, over the sheet covering the lower limbs; also,

FIG. 26.

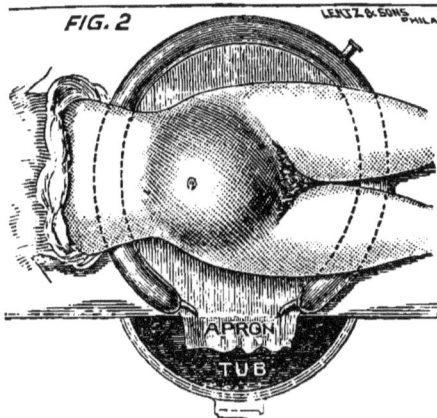

FIG. 2

LENTZ & SONS PHILA.

APRON

TUB

Arrangement of Operating Pad in Abdominal Section.

covering the rubber cloth at the sides of the patient. The dressings applied over the abdomen should not be removed until the operator is ready to proceed to his work.

Some operators prefer retaining a catheter in

7

Retention
of catheter
in bladder.
the bladder as a guide during the operation. In this case a shallow urinal or ordinary soap-dish may be slipped between the limbs to catch the urine as it flows out.

All this adjustment of clothing, protectives, etc., can be made in a very few minutes after etherization is complete.

CHAPTER IX.

PREPARATION OF OPERATOR AND ASSISTANTS.

The operator, his assistants, and nurses should be thoroughly prepared for the grave work they are to undertake by especial attention to personal cleanliness. A full bath with an entirely fresh suit of clothing, as described in the chapter on the Surgical Nurse, will be sufficient so far as concerns the general preparation of the person. The hands and arms will need further attention for their especial sterilization. The method which originated, I believe, in the Johns Hopkins Hospital and has since been employed in other institutions, has been found very satisfactory. The hands and fore-arms being thoroughly scrubbed with soap and warm water for several minutes, the finger-nails having previously been carefully cleaned and cut, the hands are immersed for about one minute in a saturated solution of permanganate of potassium, which is well rubbed into the skin. The hands are then bleached in a saturated solution of oxalic acid. The oxalic acid solution is then washed off with distilled boiled water and the

Personal cleanliness.

Methods of cleansing hands and arms.

hands finally immersed in a solution of bichloride of mercury from 1–1000 to 1–5000 for about one minute. It is claimed by the originators of this method that cultures taken from beneath the finger-nails of hands thus cleaned have been found to be absolutely sterile.

The staining effect of permanganate of potassium, which remains to some extent even after the use of oxalic acid, if the hands be thus frequently cleansed, is the chief objection to this method. It is well probably to employ it, should one be obliged to operate shortly after the handling of discharges of a foul nature. The immersion of the hands in alcohol, after a thorough cleansing with soap and water, and their subsequent immersion in a strong bichloride solution is probably sufficient for producing an antiseptic condition in ordinary cases.

Surgical aprons.

Before beginning the operation the operator and his assistants should put on long white linen aprons, enveloping the whole person, which should previously have been sterilized by steaming in the Arnold apparatus for one hour before operation, or by superheating in the sterilizing oven for a similar length of time.

Avoidance of contamination.

During the operation the surgeon and his assistants should carefully avoid touching anything that may contaminate their hands. Should they have to do so, the process of recleansing the hands should again be gone through with. A frequent dipping of the hands into the warm sterilized water provided will keep them free of blood and also conduce to greater safety in the performance of the operation.

CHAPTER X.

THE NURSE'S DUTIES DURING OPERATION.

After a careful preparation of the room and of the patient, according to the instructions laid down in the preceding chapters, the nurse will need to make the changes in her own toilet necessary to

Personal cleanliness of nurse. her attendance upon the operation. Her hands and fore-arms will need to be rendered thoroughly aseptic, and a clean apron with sleeves put on. The general bath and change of clothing should have been obtained before her preparation of the patient.

Arrangement of patient for operation. When ready herself the nurse should assist in taking the patient into the operating room, placing her on the table and arranging the clothing and protectives. After doing this, if she is not otherwise directed by the surgeon in attendance, she can see to arranging such details as have had to be left to the last; as placing sterilized water of the proper temperature in the various vessels provided for the purposes of irrigation, cleansing of sponges and hands, etc. A good temperature to start with is 110° or 115° Fahr.

She should see that hot bottles or foot-warmers Warming of bed. are placed in the bed which is to receive the patient after operation. She should take a careful survey of the room and see that everything is in its proper place, that is, where it may be most readily obtained when wanted.

After assuring herself that all is right, she should Management of sponges. recleanse her hands and take up her station at the stand where she is to manage the sponges.

As rapidly as the soiled sponges are thrown into the cold-water basin, she should cleanse them of blood, rinse them out of the hot water, and place them in the basin on the stand to the assistant's right.

She should keep her eyes open to the needs of Special duties. the operator and his assistants, supplying sponges, clean towels, etc., as needed ; keeping the water in the various basins changed as it becomes soiled, and finally assisting with the removal of the soiled clothing, the application of dressings, and the removal of the patient to the bed. While the surgeon is completing his application of the dressings the Preparation of bed for reception of patient. nurse should turn back the covers from the bed, and remove the hot-water bottles, etc., temporarily, placing them under the bed to be out of the way until the patient has been placed in bed, when they may be replaced around her.

The nurse's hands should be frequently cleansed

as she passes from one thing to another in her attention to the various details of service.

When the patient has been placed in bed and warmly covered with blankets, the hot applications being placed around her, a towel should be placed under her chin, a light basin under the head of the bed to be on hand should she vomit, and a towel wrung out of cold water may be placed upon her forehead. The blinds or screens.should be so arranged that the light in the room may be modified. A chair for the surgeon may be placed at the head of the bed, and, as he or his assistant takes his place there, the nurse may attend to

speedily removing the things used during the operation, as tables, protectives, etc., from the room. These may be placed temporarily in an adjoining room, until the nurse or some one who volunteers to assist her may see the different articles taken back to their respective places in the house.

Sheets, etc., soiled with blood, should be placed in a tub to soak. This will render the washing of them quite easy, as the blood being well-rinsed out of them, they may then be placed in the ordinary wash, unless it is preferred to do them separately.

Screens being placed around the bed to prevent the patient's feeling the draught, the windows should be raised and doors opened to thoroughly change the air in the apartment. This may more effectually be done by "pumping the door," as it is called, that is rapidly opening and closing it, without latching, so as to use it as a fan as it swings upon its hinges.

When the surgeon has to leave the patient, the nurse must take up her station by the bed. Like a sentinel on duty, she should be vigilant in her watch, noting every symptom promptly and meeting its demands. Until the patient is well out of ether the nurse should not entrust her care, even for a moment, to any inexperienced person.

The nurse's watch over patient's condition.

CHAPTER XI.

THE NURSE'S DUTIES AFTER OPERATION AND DURING CONVALESCENCE.

The immediate duties of the nurse after operation will depend much upon the condition in which the patient has been put to bed.

Treatment of shock. If the condition of shock be profound, vigorous measures may be necessary to produce a reaction. The application of dry heat, by means of blankets heated in an oven and tucked closely around the patient, and of pieces of flannel heated and placed over the chest immediately next the skin, serves to stimulate the circulation. The extremities may be rubbed with whiskey or brandy, the nurse's hands being carried under the blankets to avoid exposure to air. The head should be kept low, even lower than the feet, in order to keep up the circulation of blood in the brain. The foot of the bed may be elevated for this purpose, being raised by means of bricks or stools, or a high chair upon which a stool has been placed may be slipped under the foot-board.

The patient may be fanned, and hartshorn sprinkled on a handkerchief or towel held near the

nostrils. Should further measures be necessary
the nurse may, with the sanction of the surgeon,
give hypodermic injections of some stimulant.
Brandy or whisky may be thus given, or solutions
of caffeine, strychnia, or digitalis. These are intended to strengthen the heart's action, and, if
doing their work properly, the effect should be soon
noted in the pulse. It should grow stronger and
slower. The frequency with which these injections
should be given and the amount given at one time,
will in every case need to be regulated by the surgeon. Careful instructions must be obtained from
him. The full 30 minims of brandy or whisky
may be given, filling the barrel of the syringe full.
Ten to fifteen minims of tincture of digitalis generally constitutes a dose. It may be diluted in
sufficient water to fill the barrel of the syringe. One
to two grains of caffeine in solution, or $\frac{1}{60}$ gr. of
strychnia in solution, may be given by computing
the dose according to the strength of the solution
compounded.

Hypoder-
mic use of
stimulants
in shock.

The hypodermic syringe is a delicate instrument
and should be carefully managed and kept in good
order, so that it may be ready for use at any time.
The barrel may be of metal, glass, or rubber ; the
nozzle or needle of gold, silver, or steel. The
latter should be very sharp, hence the point should
be kept well protected. If dulled its introduction

Care of hy-
podermic
syringe.

will cause pain. After use, a fine gold wire should be run through it, from the point of the needle upward, to keep out dust, etc.   The barrel should be kept filled ⅓ full of water to keep the packing of the piston soft. Should the packing become loose, draw out the piston and slip the fingernail around the upper part of the packing, and spread it a little and soak in a little warm water for a time. A screw-piece attached to the piston enables a more

FIG. 27.

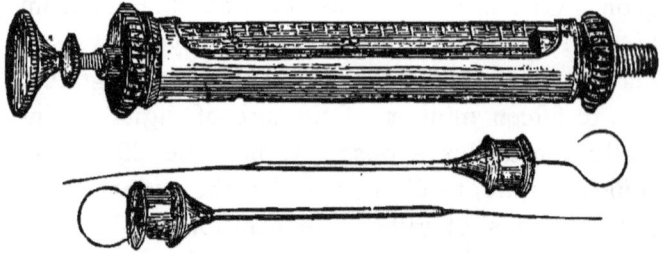

Hypodermic Needles and Syringe.

accurate regulation of the dose, when it has to be estimated in minims.   In administering the injec-

Method of hypoder-mic injec-tion.

tion take hold of a portion of the upper part of the arm or thigh and hold it firmly for a little time to benumb sensation ; then insert the needle quickly, but not too deeply, straight down into this mass and carefully inject the fluid. After withdrawing the needle put your finger over the point from which it was withdrawn, and rub over the place for a little time to prevent any of the fluid coming back.

When the patient's strength is low, stimulating or nutrient enemata are often given. For simple stimulation a gill of black coffee, strained and carefully injected into the bowel, is excellent. Stimulating or nutrient enemata.

As a feeding enema, milk, beef-tea, broth, etc., alone or combined with stimulants, may be employed. All feeding enemata should be peptonized to render their digestion and assimilation easier, for there is but little digestive power in the lower bowel.

The amount given to an adult at one time should not exceed 1 gill, and should not be given oftener than once in 3 or 4 hours. It is better to give highly concentrated food, rather than to give these injections too frequently, for the bowel is thus irritated and will not retain the food given.

A tablespoonful of expressed beef-juice, which represents the nutriment from ¼ pound of beef, may be combined with a gill of warm water, to which whisky or brandy may be added from 1 teaspoonful to 1 tablespoonful, according to the surgeon's desire.

This given once in 3 hours will represent considerable nourishment. Medication may be combined with the food thus given, as 15–20 drops tincture of digitalis or aromatic spirits of ammonia.

The injection should be given at a temperature
of 100° Fahr. If too warm or too cold, it will
stimulate the action of the bowels.

An ordinary Davidson hand-ball syringe may be
used as a siphon for the introduction of this enema
from the cup containing it. Care should be taken
to inject no air into the bowel. It is well to introduce a vaginal nozzle into the bowel a few minutes

FIG. 28.

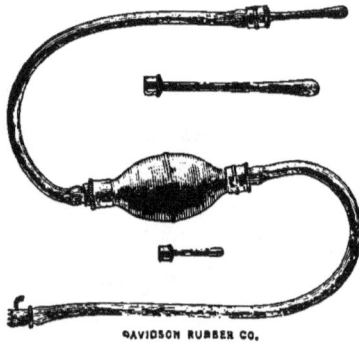

Davidson Syringe.

before the time for giving the enema, to allow of the
escape of any gas that may have collected and
thus better insure the retention of the food. A
bowel used thus for purposes of nutrition should
be washed out at least once daily, to remove any
residue that may collect and prevent ready absorption. This may be done by injecting a pint of warm

water in which has been dissolved a teaspoonful of salt. If this is not voluntarily evacuated a nozzle may be inserted to draw it off. To administer the stimulating enema itself, all air is first expelled from the syringe by keeping the ends beneath the surface of the mixture and compressing the bulb until no bubbles are produced. A little vaseline may then be used to anoint the nozzle, which is then carefully insinuated into the bowel. If the direction of the lower bowel is remembered by the nurse as first extending for a short distance toward the vagina and then inclining backward, there will be no difficulty experienced in introducing the nozzle without causing any pain. The nozzle must then be held in place. The patient, if strong enough, can do this for herself, and the nurse will raise the vessel containing the mixture to be injected. As soon as the last of the liquid flows into the syringe, the tubing should be compressed while the nozzle is withdrawn. This is to prevent the introduction of air into the bowel. A napkin may then be held Method of firmly applied for a time to the anus, until the insuring re-tention. irritability of the bowel ceases.

The addition of white of egg beaten into the mixture, or a teaspoonful of starch or arrowroot, will serve to make the liquid injected less irritating to the bowel. When the bowel becomes non-retentive the addition of from 10 to 15 drops of laudanum to the enema may enable it to be retained. Opium in any form should not be used without the express direction of the surgeon. If preferred, a barrel and piston syringe may be used in giving these injections.

The precaution should be taken to inject the fluid very slowly.

Period in which danger from hemorrhage; from inflammation; from blood-poisoning.

The greatest danger in the first twenty-four hours after operation is from hemorrhage; in the first three or four days from inflammation; and the first ten days from blood-poisoning. The nurse should look frequently at the dressings and the clothing under the patient's back to see if there be any bleeding.

Symptoms of internal hemorrhage.

If there is internal bleeding it will show itself by the patient being faint, white or blue around the lips, and the pulse becoming very faint and rapid, or else altogether lost. Hemorrhage occurring in the first twenty-four to forty eight hours after operation is called primary hemorrhage. Secondary hemorrhage comes on generally in the second week.

Primary hemorrhage.

Secondary hemorrhage.

Reaction after operation.

Reaction after operation is shown by the patient's speaking, the pulse getting stronger and the skin becoming moist and warm. When this occurs it is undesirable to keep up too much artificial heat about the patient. The heated bottles, etc., around her may therefore be removed.

The temperature, pulse, and respiration of the patient should be taken immediately after she is placed in bed, and after that every 3 hours for the first few days. The temperature is best taken in the arm-pit. Record of temperature, etc.

For the sake of uniformity it is well to make the record of temperature, pulse, etc., come at 12, 3, 6, and 9 o'clock. Special symptoms to be noted.

The nurse should note all symptoms accurately and report them carefully. If the patient is uneasy or complains of pain, note this down in the record. If she is sick or vomits, report the time, quantity, and appearance of the matter vomited.

During any retching or vomiting the nurse should place one hand over the site of the wound, to prevent undue strain upon the stitches or the forcing out of the drainage tube.

The quieter the patient is kept the better, therefore no conversation should go on in the room. Do not let the patient lift her head or move her limbs. Report chills or chilliness. Give just as little nourishment as possible for the first few days, unless directed otherwise by the surgeon.

The ordinary rule for feeding after a laparotomy is as follows :— Management of diet.

For first 24 hours absolutely nothing, not even ice or water. If the lips and mouth are much parched with ether, a small soft piece of linen cloth

8

may be dipped in cold water and used to moisten the mouth and tongue.

If the stomach is settled the patient may on the second day take a teaspoonful of barley water every hour. If this is retained she may on the third day have a teaspoonful of milk combined with the barley water. When the bowels have been once thoroughly moved, as they should be by the third day, the dietary may be increased. The food at first should be concentrated rather than large in quantity. As the amount is increased the intervals should be lengthened, thus, a tablespoonful of expressed beef-juice may be given alternating with a tablespoonful of milk once in two hours.

Should the liquid diet tend to produce flatulence, bread-crumbs may be used with the milk and beef-juice, or a partial semi-liquid diet may be substituted; thus, farina, junket, wheat-germ, thickened milk, koumiss, toast milk, wine whey, strained gruel, rice, milk-toast, broths containing rice or barley may gradually be substituted. By the close of the second week the patient may gradually resume ordinary, plain, wholesome fare. The occasional use of a baked apple, or a dish of stewed apples, will aid in regulating the bowels. Should the patient's stomach be retentive and her general condition good, an occasional drink of very weak, hot tea, in place of the barley water, on the second and third days will be found, by relieving the feeling of exhaustion, to steady the nerves and add to the patient's comfort. For the control of vomiting various devices have been recommended. Control of vomiting.

As the vomiting after ether is largely the result of cerebral congestion, it is desirable to keep the head cool by the application of cloths wrung out in ice water or icebags. This relieves also the accompanying headache.

A mustard-paste placed over the stomach will be sedative in its effect upon the vomiting. Should the tendency continue notwithstanding this treatment, a feeder full of very hot water containing a small pinch of salt, may be sipped by the patient. This will probably come up, but will serve to quiet the tendency to retching. Another means which is often effectual is that of injecting about ½ pint of warm water (105° Fahr.) into the rectum and having it retained.

Intestinal colic is frequently complained of, especially during the second and third day. It is caused by the accumulation of gas in the intestines. Intestinal colic.
There is apt to be such an accumulation in the large bowel, just below the diaphragm, causing the patient often to cry out with pain. The use of a warm flaxseed poultice over this region will relieve the pain and enable the gas to work down into the lower bowel. The use of the vaginal nozzle in the

rectum will enable it often to be expelled and thus relieve the pain.   The drink of hot tea or very hot water will also aid in this result.

The nurse should learn from the surgeon what his desire may be concerning the use of the catheter. Unless especial directions are given the catheter may be used once in six hours.

After hysterectomy it may be necessary to empty the bladder once in every three or four hours, if the stump is so situated as to interfere with its

FIG. 29.

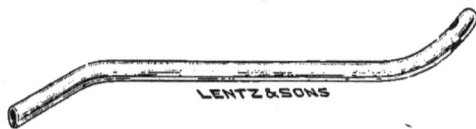

Glass Catheter.

proper distention.   The silver or glass catheter should be used, or the soft rubber catheter.   Great care should be exercised by thorough cleanliness to produce no irritation from its use.   The instruments, if glass or silver, should be boiled after each use, and kept in the intervals in a weak solution 1–40 of carbolic acid.   The part around the orifice of the urethra should be carefully cleansed before the insertion of the catheter.   The catheter itself should be well lubricated with a little carbolized vaseline.

It is probably best to insert the catheter by sight, the efforts to do it by touch, unless one is especially skilled, often inducing irritation.   The patient may be so protected by the covers that but little exposure is necessary in its use, a blanket or sheet being thrown over each limb, the urinal being placed between them.   Should the nurse be able to use the catheter by touch, the operation can be performed without any exposure beneath the covers. The index finger of the nurse's right hand should

FIG. 30.

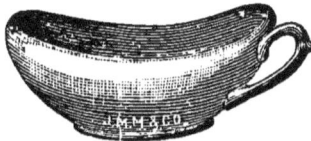

Coach Urinal.

be slipped into the vagina as far as the second joint, and made to follow the anterior vaginal wall down in the median line to the vaginal entrance, when a little elevation of the surface will be felt, immediately above which the orifice of the urethra is to be found.   If the finger be held with its palmar surface upward and resting lightly upon this elevation, the finger being held horizontally, a catheter slipped along it will enter the small orifice of the urethra.   Should the extremity of the catheter seem to meet with any obstruction after its entrance into the urethra, a slight withdrawal and rotation of the instrument will generally carry it in. After the catheter has been withdrawn the parts should be cleansed and dried.

Urinals.

Should the patient be allowed to pass her own water, the tin slipper urinal or the china or glass urinal made to fit over the vulva may be employed. Should there be difficulty in urination, fomentations applied over the vulva, or hot water in the urinal or bedpan will sometimes aid its accomplishment.

FIG. 31.

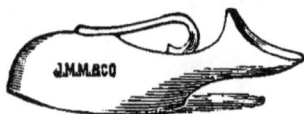

Female Urinal of China or Glass.

Notes concerning character of urine.

The urine drawn should be measured and tested with litmus paper, and a note made on the record of its amount, appearance, and reaction. If there is anything peculiar in its appearance, that is, if it is smoky or bloody, or contains sediment, save it for the surgeon's inspection at his next visit.

Saving of napkins for inspection.

The same should be done with napkins containing any discharge that may come from the vagina, and the fact should be reported on the nurse's record.

Report also any cough; state what kind it was —tight or loose—how long it lasted. Report hiccoughs. Report also the character of the sleep, as heavy, quiet, uneasy, or if the patient snores. Report if the patient complains of the bandages feeling tight, for inflammation is shown by the distention of the abdomen. Report any change that may be seen in the patient, and send the doctor word concerning it, if it is at all serious. The temperature of the room should be kept at from 68° to 70°. It should not be allowed to vary. The patient should be carefully kept from all draughts, but thorough ventilation of the apartment should be obtained. Screens carefully adjusted enable this to be accomplished. All discharges, wash water, etc., should be at once removed from the room. The slop-jar for the wash water should not stand in the sick-room, but in an adjoining room.

Report of cough, etc.

Temperature of room.

Hygienic precautions.

After an evacuation of the bowels especial care should be taken to change the air of the apartment. The bedpan should always be carefully covered in its removal to the water-closet. A newspaper or napkin may be thrown over it, if it has no cover of its own.

An early evacuation of the bowels is very desirable after an abdominal section. The exact period will be dependent upon the patient's condition. Should all go well and the patient suffer

Method of securing an evacuation of bowels after operation.

little from flatulence, it is not necessary to make any effort to have the bowels moved before the third day. At that time means should be taken to have a movement with as little straining as possible. A rectal injection of a gill of cotton-seed or sweet-oil with a tablespoonful of turpentine may be given, and should be retained, if possible, about two hours, when a soap-and-water injection may be given.

A very good method of securing a movement is by the enema composed of Epsom salts, oil, turpentine and glycerine combined with water, which has already been mentioned in the chapter on Preparation of the Patient.

This enema is almost always followed by an immediate evacuation of the bowels.

After this has been secured, any irritability of the bowel that may ensue, may be allayed by the injection of about 1 gill of warm water containing a little table salt in solution. This is to be retained.

Administration of salts by mouth.

Should enemata fail to secure a satisfactory evacuation, salts may be administered by mouth. A teaspoonful of Rochelle salts may be given dissolved in a tablespoonful of hot water, and followed by a few sips of hot water. This dose may be repeated every hour, should the patient retain it, until from four to six doses have been taken or the bowels feel like moving. This followed by the use of a simple soap-sud enema will, as a rule, have the desired effect. The salts are best administered in this concentrated form when it is desired to secure prompt effect. The nauseating effect of the dose may be avoided by a little circumspection in its administration. The solution of the salts should be placed in one feeder, and the hot water to be sipped, in a separate feeder. The patient should be directed to put the spout of the feeder as far back in her mouth as she can, and to swallow the salts quickly, not allowing any to touch the tip of the tongue and the lips, where the sense of taste is

FIG. 32.

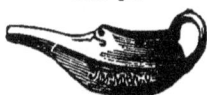

Feeder.

strongest. She may follow this immediately with the sips of hot water from the feeder on hand. The nurse should place her hand beneath the pillow and slightly raise the head of the patient in giving her anything to swallow. A napkin should be placed beneath the chin to prevent spilling on the clothing. This rule for administration should be followed in giving food as well as medicine.

The use of the bedpan involves considerable risk to the patient unless great care is used in lifting her. Particularly is this true in cases of hys- *Use of bedpan. Methods of employing.*

terectomy, when there is greater danger from the occurrence of hemorrhage or from formation of clots in the blood-vessels. The nurse should not attempt to perform this duty alone, unless she is

FIG. 33.

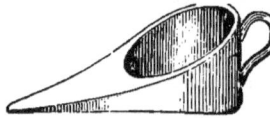

Slipper Bed-Pan.

fully equal to lifting the patient without jarring. Should the patient be slight and of light weight, the nurse may place one arm under the patient's knees, slightly lifting the hips. With the other hand the bedpan may be slipped under them.

FIG. 34.

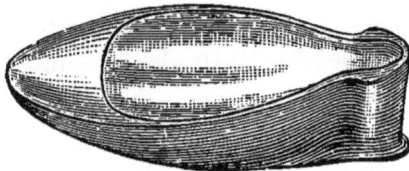

Eureka Bed-Pan.

Should the patient be heavy, she is better lifted by placing one hand under each hip and slightly raising her thus from above. Another attendant can then slip the pan under. The same manœuvre should be resorted to in removing the pan.

Should the patient be too feeble or the nurse unable to get the proper help, the tin-slipper urinal is a convenient receptacle to use, and will involve no lifting. It is well to have two of these to use interchangeably, because of their small size.

Should the nurse not have these, she may use pads made of newspaper and soft rags or oakum, which can be worked under the patient without any lifting, and which, after use, can be simply rolled up and burned. The amount and character of the movement should be carefully recorded on the report, as also should the fact as to the expulsion of gas from the bowel at any time. *Pads as substitutes for bedpans.* *Particulars to be reported.*

The patient should be scrupulously cleaned after these movements, and the parts kept thoroughly dry. Especial care should be taken to see that there is no moisture under the back and that the skin is kept from breaking. The surface upon which the patient lies should be perfectly smooth. Wrinkles tend to produce sores. Bedsores may develop in so short a time as the result of pressure and moisture that a nurse must exercise the greatest vigilance in their prevention. Rubbing the back daily at least once or twice with a little alcohol and alum serves to harden the skin. This may be followed by rubbing with powdered oxide of zinc or starch or bismuth subnitrate as a drying powder. *Prevention of bedsores.*

When the skin has broken the treatment must be

changed.   Some ointment will be necessary to
soothe and heal the raw surface.   The alcohol and
alum, if used, would cause pain and irritation.
Borated or carbolized zinc ointment applied on lint
and held on with adhesive strips will constitute the
best dressing.   A most important feature of treatment is relief from pressure.   A ring cushion of

FIG. 35.

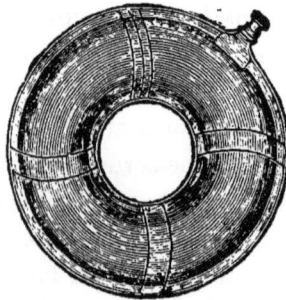

Rubber Air-Cushion.

rubber may be used for this purpose, being placed
beneath the patient in such a way that the bedsore
shall rest over the hole in the ring.   When a rubber cushion cannot be had the nurse may make a
circular cushion of the kind, filling it with soft rags
or hair.

Location of
bedsores.   Bedsores may come on any part of the body
which is subjected to pressure, as the shoulder, the
elbows, the lower part of the back and the heels.

The skin over the sacrum, or end of the backbone is probably the most frequent site for such a sore.

Skill in the management of a drainage tube is one of the most important qualifications on the part of the nurse. The methods employed by different operators vary somewhat, hence the nurse must

Fig. 36.

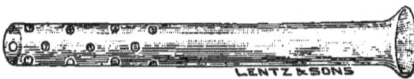

Glass Drainage Tube.

obtain explicit directions from the surgeon in charge of a case.

The intervals may be, according to his choice, from once every half hour to once in twelve hours or more.

Fig. 37.

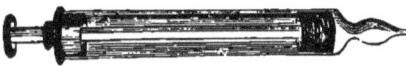

Glass Syringe for Draining Tube.

Draining of the tube by means of a syringe Method of draining. may be accomplished either with the barrel and piston syringe of glass or hard rubber, to which a piece of rubber tubing is attached, or by what is known as the hard-rubber uterine syringe with long nozzle. These syringes should be kept in the intervals of use in an antiseptic solution, as 1–4000 bichloride of mercury. The sponge taken from over the drainage tube should be put in a weak carbolic solution until again wanted. A small glass graduate is convenient for receiving the fluid drawn from the tube and accurately recording its amount.

In making preparations for draining, the nurse should first arrange the covers over the patient's chest and over the lower limbs, so that just the portion of the body covered by the abdominal

FIG. 38.

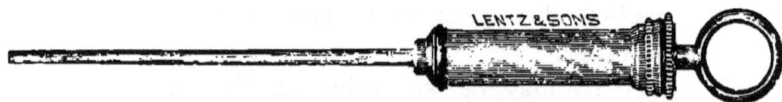

Hard Rubber Syringe for Draining Tube.

bandage shall be exposed to view. She shall then thoroughly cleanse her hands, rendering them aseptic and loosen the bandage and rubber dressing. Again washing off her hands in an antiseptic solution, she should lay back the rubber covering of the tube, remove the sponge, closing over its orifice, placing it in a carbolized solution, and take up the syringe with which she is going to drain the tube. The rubber tubing or the nozzle is allowed carefully to slip down through the glass drainage tube into the abdomen. If the extremity of the tube is felt to meet with a point of resistance, it should be drawn back a little before suction is effected by drawing on the handle of the syringe. The syringe should be very carefully and slowly filled and then drawn out. A corner of the rubber protective may be thrown over the mouth of the tube until the syringe is emptied and rinsed out. The contents of the syringe may be emptied into the glass graduate provided. The use of the syringe is continued until no liquid remains. The sponge is then squeezed out of the carbolic solution and replaced over the drainage tube. The corners of the rubber protective are folded back over the sponge and pinned, and the bandage, if need be, readjusted. The liquid drained should be placed in a small labeled bottle—of which a number should be prepared before the operation—and the date and hour with the record of the amount drained should be placed on the label. This enables the surgeon to obtain an accurate idea of the character of the drainage.

When the hard rubber syringe is used care must be taken not to jar the sides of the drainage tube. Unless the syringe works easily this is apt to be done. The suction also may be so strong that portions of omentum or bowel may be drawn into the tube through its perforations.

Capillary
drainage.

A third method of draining is by what is known as capillary drainage; a twist of sterilized cotton or gauze is placed down into the drainage tube and sucks up the liquid. The dressing over the mouth of the tube thus becomes saturated and requires changing. Some surgeons like the tube cleansed by means of small tampons of sterilized cotton, carried down into it by means of a long, slender pair of forceps, very like the uterine dressing forceps. A new twist of cotton is then placed in the tube. The amount of fluid drained should be recorded on the nurse's report, and its character described each time. When the liquid becomes pale, losing its bloody hue, it is pure serum, and the surgeon will probably desire to remove the tube. The nurse will need to prepare a basin containing bichloride solution, about 1–4000, for the doctor's hands, and another with carbolic solution, 1–40, for the instruments (scissors and forceps) which may be used. A tray containing fresh dressings and adhesive strips should also be ready. When the stitches are to be removed, which is usually during the second week, similar preparations should be made.

Bathing
after opera-
tion.

The advisability of bathing the patient during her convalescence should be determined by the surgeon. The cleansing previous to operation having been so very thorough, it is, as a rule, unnecessary to give a full sponge bath and change the clothing for about one week after. It would probably involve too much moving of the patient. The head, neck, chest, hands and arms may be sponged separately as occasion may call for it. The same may be done with the lower extremities. This is less exhausting than the general bath at one time. With sufficient care the patient's cloth- Changing of clothing. ing may be changed without moving her too much. This can only be done properly if the precaution has been taken to have the clothing very loose. In removing the nightdress and undervest, the sleeves should be slipped off on one side, and the arm and shoulder covered by a blanket. They may be then taken off the opposite side in the same way. The sleeves of the fresh undervest having been drawn through the sleeves of the fresh night-dress, the two garments may be slipped on at once. The sleeves of one side may be drawn on and then those of the opposite side. An assistant slipping her hands under the shoulders and slightly raising them, the nurse may draw out the soiled clothing from beneath the back, and slip the neck of the fresh undervest and nightdress over the patient's head, drawing the garments well down and smooth-ing out all wrinkles under the back. The sleeves also should be straightened, so that there may be no feeling of constriction under the armpit. The

9

drawers may be changed without much moving, as it is not necessary to draw them under the back and fasten them.

The abdominal bandage and dressings can be better managed when the drawers are allowed to remain as a loose covering for the limbs. The change of stockings involves no disturbance of the patient. Greater difficulty will be experienced in changing the bedclothing beneath the patient. If the draw-sheet is kept carefully changed and the covers, a change of the other bedclothing may be deferred—unless in case of accident—until the second week. To change the draw-sheet, unpin it from its fastenings and pin one end of the fresh draw-sheet, properly folded, to one end of the sheet to be removed.

As the hips of the patient are slightly raised by the nurse, the soiled draw-sheet can be quickly drawn out and the new one drawn under the patient by an assistant on the other side of the bed. The fresh draw-sheet may then be unpinned from the soiled one and its ends tucked under the mattress and pinned.

The pillow will need to be removed, beaten, turned and the slips changed quite frequently. The comfort of the patient is greatly increased by an occasional turning and adjustment of the pillows.

If two beds have been provided to be used

interchangeably during the patient's convalescence, the change may be easily effected by lifting the patient from one bed into another.   It is necessary to have three persons to do this without jarring. All three should stand on the same side of the bed, the tallest nearest to the patient's head, the shortest nearest the feet. The attendant nearest the head should place one arm under the patient's neck, so that the head may lie upon it, and gain a secure hold with the hand of the same arm under the axilla on the opposite side of her. The other arm should be extended just below the shoulder blades.

The second attendant places one arm under the small of the back and the other arm just below the buttocks. The third assistant places one arm under the knees and the other under the ankle. When all three have their arms properly adjusted, a signal—" Now !"—may be given by one of them, and all must lift simultaneously.

This will enable the patient to be raised without the slightest jar and transferred to the new bed. The latter should have been placed conveniently near, the covers folded back, and the pillow placed so that it will be at the right end of the bed for the patient's head when the nurses turn around in lifting her from the one bed to the other.

When two beds cannot be had, the least disturbance is probably produced in the changing of

the bedclothing by unfastening the undersheet or
blanket and the draw-sheet upon which the patient
lies, rolling them up from one side of the bed close
to the patient, adjusting a fresh draw-sheet to a
fresh undersheet, rolling them up lengthwise and
spreading so far as possible over the uncovered
side of the bed, tucking them under the mattress at
the side. The remainder of the two sheets is gathered into a roll and carried close up to the roll
made by the soiled clothing. If the patient can be
turned on her side, both these rolls may then be
carried well under her as she turns on the opposite
side, and in turning back she will turn over them,
thus enabling both the soiled clothing and the fresh
to be carried through to the opposite side and
properly adjusted to the bed, the soiled clothing
being removed. Should it be considered unwise
to let the patient roll on her side, her hips may be
slightly lifted and the rolls of soiled and fresh
clothing drawn through by an assistant who stands
on the opposite side. The same manœuvre can be
carried out with the shoulders and the lower extremities until the fresh clothing is properly arranged.

Another method is that of drawing the patient
well to one side of the bed on the sheet upon which
she lies. The fresh sheets may then be placed
over the rest of the bed and gathered into a roll

close to the patient's side.   The patient may then be lifted or drawn over on to the fresh sheets.   The old sheet may be gradually removed from under her and the remaining portion of the fresh sheets unrolled and spread over the uncovered portion of the bed.

The covers can be changed by spreading the fresh sheet and blanket over the former covering, and working the latter down to the foot of the bed beneath these, thus removing them.

The limbs of the patient frequently become be- Massage numbed and ache for want of exercise.   The nurse for passive exercise. may help this by rubbing them and gently kneading the muscles from time to time.   It is not necessary to remove the clothing for this.   There is generally no objection to slightly bending the limbs at the knees and supporting them on a pillow. Small pillows, 6 inches wide and 8 to 12 long, made of hair, are convenient for placing around the patient to remove pressure and produce slight changes in the position which are restful.

Before sitting up the patient should be fitted with Necessity for abdomi- a bandage for the support of the abdominal walls. nal sup-porter. As a rule, this bandage should be worn for one year, being removed only at night or when the patient lies down.   This is to prevent rupture at the site of the incision.   The bandage usually employed in the " Woman's Hospital " is that known

as the London Supporter. A modification of this
has been employed in cases of long incision reach-
ing above the umbilicus. When there is not much
strain upon the abdominal walls the ordinary elastic abdominal bandage serves the purpose very
nicely. Great circumspection should be employed
regarding the patient's sitting up after she has sufficiently convalesced to do so.

FIG. 39.

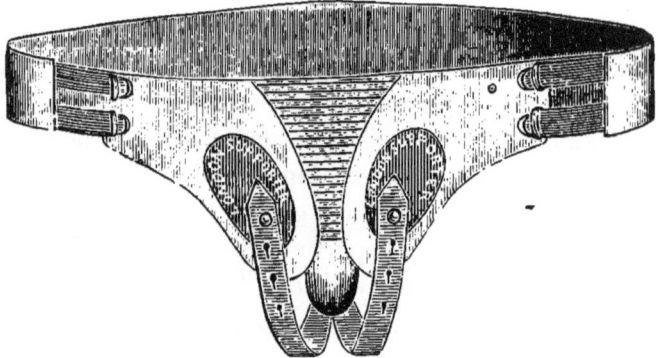

London Supporter.

The first
sitting-up.

The period at first should be short. It is better
to lift the patient out on a sofa or reclining chair
for a change, rather than allow her to overexert
herself. The surgeon should be carefully consulted
as to the amount and character of the exercise the
patient may take.

The general directions given in this chapter may

be greatly modified by different surgeons. The nurse must be prepared to respond to the requirements of the surgeon in every case. A nurse should never let it be known that her views differ Code of ethics in nursing.

FIG. 40.

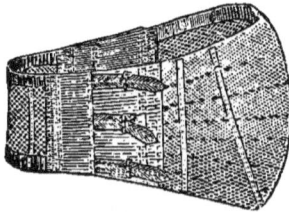

Elastic Abdominal Bandage.

from those of her superior officer. It is right always for the surgeon or physician to plan the campaign in the management of a case. The nurse, if she serves under him, has but one duty—to obey.

CHAPTER XII.

MANAGEMENT OF COMPLICATIONS.

Signifi-
cance of rise
of tempera-
ture. *Rise of Temperature.*—This symptom always should cause anxiety after an operation, especially when the temperature exceeds 102° Fahr., for it is so frequently the indication of blood-poisoning in one or another form. The rise, however, may be due to some other cause, as a cold, bronchitis, ague, or it may denote the approach of a menstrual period, or may accompany a discharge from the uterus, which is not infrequent a few days after operation upon the pelvic organs. Extreme excitement may similarly produce an elevation of the temperature for a time. The treatment of this fever must depend largely upon the cause.

Means for
reduction
of tempera-
ture. When the temperature rises above 102° and there is a similar increase in the pulse, some means should be taken for its reduction. An ice-cap may be placed upon the head and should be kept on until the temperature has steadily gone down, remaining below 100°. The face, hands, and wrists may be frequently sponged with cold water. Wet-packing is sometimes employed where the temper-

ature keeps very high, notwithstanding the ice-cap.

The arms may first be packed in wet towels, wrung out in ice-cold water, and kept moist by water squeezed upon them from a sponge. The lower extremities and the chest may require the same treatment, if the application of cold to the arms fails to reduce the temperature. A rubber protective will need to be slipped under the patient when this treatment is carried out, to prevent wetting of the bedclothing.

An icebag is sometimes directed to be placed over the heart for the reduction of temperature. When these means are employed the pulse and temperature must be frequently taken, as great depression may occur suddenly. The necessity for keeping a patient very still will prevent the use of the fever-cot in the early days after operation. Later, however, it may be employed. No heroic measures, such as the above, should, however, be employed without the full sanction of the surgeon. The use of antipyretic remedies will also be directed by him.

The ice-cap ordinarily employed in this country is a simple rubber bag, which is filled one-third full of pieces of ice about the size of a walnut. All air should then be squeezed out of the bag and a piece of string fastened securely around the neck. The

Sudden depression from application of cold.

Fever-cot.

Ice-cap.

bag is then placed on top of the patient's head, a single layer of muslin or toweling intervening between them. If the bag is filled more than one-third full it will not adapt itself well to the shape of the head. Two bags should be in use at the same time, so that the nurse may have one to immediately replace the other when refilling of the bag is necessary. The ice melts so fast when the fever is high that the bag will probably need refilling about every 20 minutes or half hour. It is utterly useless for the purpose of reducing temperature after the ice has melted.

Noiseless method for cracking ice.

The nurse will need to have ice close at hand for the purpose. A block wrapped in flannel and kept in a covered vessel in a cool part of the room, or in the adjoining hall, will enable her to keep up this application without much difficulty. With a large steel pin and with the piece of ice wrapped in a cloth the nurse may noiselessly break off the pieces required for filling the cap. The pin pressed firmly into the ice will cause it to separate into pieces, which can similarly be broken into smaller pieces if desired. When the rubber icebag cannot be had, a pig's bladder, obtained at a drug store for ten cents, serves the purpose very well, although it is more perishable.

Leiter's tubes.

Pliable metal coils, through which cold water may be made to circulate continuously, are some-

times used for reduction of temperature. These
are called Leiter's tubes. They may be adapted

FIG. 41.

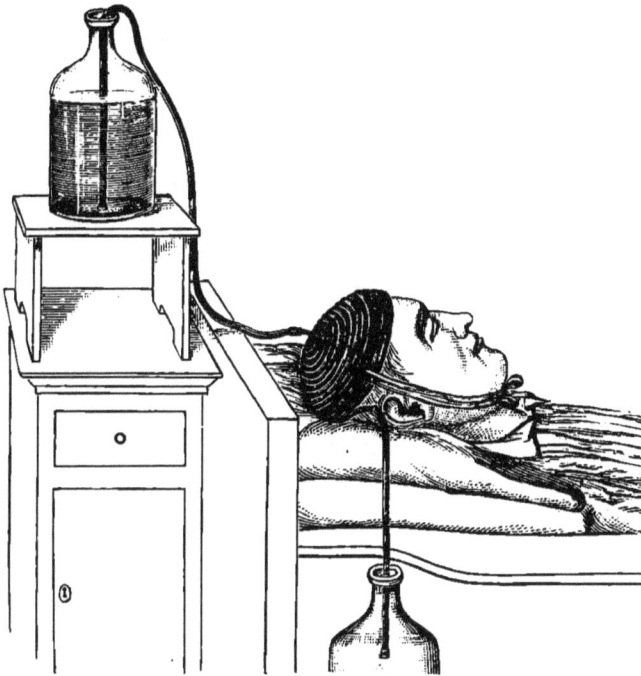

Leiter's Tube Cap.

for application to various parts of the body. The
coils forming a cap are used for application to the
head.

Method of application of ice-cap. A broad tape fastened under the chin holds the cap to the head. A reservoir containing the ice water is placed above the level of the patient's head and is connected by a piece of rubber tubing with the coils. A similar tube connected with the other end of the coils is placed in a receiving vessel on the floor. A slight suction made on the lower tube either by the mouth or by means of a barrel and piston syringe, establishes the siphon action. When the lower vessel is nearly full the position of the two vessels may be reversed. This continuous flow of water through the spiral cap may be kept up any length of time required. The water in the supply vessel should contain ice.

Leiter's temperature regulator. Some surgeons use by preference Leiter's temperature regulator, a long and narrow set of coils, which may be bent so as to shape it to the back and sides of the head. It is thought that better results are obtained by the application of cold to this portion of the head.

To mould these coils they should be bent over some firm convex surface, as the thigh, for, if bent by the hands, the coils will not lie parallel and they will be apt to become leaky. This regulator is connected in the same way as the cap with the supply and receiving vessels.

Water-coils of rubber. Thornton's icecap consists of a series of coils of stout gutta-percha tubing, joined together so as to

form a cap. The tubing is flat on the inner side, so
that a uniformly cool, smooth surface touches the
patient's head.   At the top of the cap one end of
the tubing is connected with a pail filled with water
containing ice.   The tubing at the lower border of
the cap terminates in a long free end which passes
from the side of the patient's head into a bucket
beside the bed.

The pail supplying the water is fitted with a top

FIG. 42.

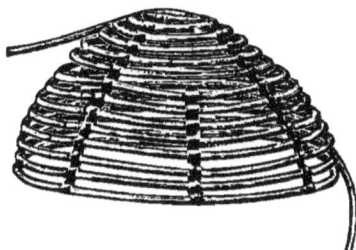

Rubber Water-coil.

which may be regulated so as to allow the water to
flow slowly.

As the receiving pail fills, the water may be baled
out and returned to the pail above.   The ice must
be kept supplied in the upper pail.   Care must be
taken in the use of the cap to see that the free tubing does not bend at an angle at any point and so
obstruct the flow or escape of water.

Fever re-
ducer.

A device consisting of a metallic reservoir for ice which surrounds the head—at a distance of a few inches from it—thus producing a layer of cool air around it, has been used to some extent in this country, particularly in the west. It is the invention of Mr. Edwin B. Magill, of South Bend, Washington, and is said to have afforded good results in practice. It is called a " fever reducer " or " body cooler."

Septi-
cæmia.

Septicæmia, Pyæmia, Peritonitis.—Septicæmia is a diseased or poisoned condition of the blood produced by absorption of putrid matter.

Pyæmia is a similar condition produced by purulent infection.

Peritonitis.

Peritonitis is inflammation of the peritoneum.

The relations between septicæmia and peritonitis appear to be very close.

Symptoms
of peri-
tonitis.

The characteristic symptoms of the latter are violent pains in the abdomen, increased by the slightest pressure, often by simple weight of the bedclothes, the pulse becoming very rapid and wiry. The temperature is not correspondingly increased, although somewhat elevated. These symptoms of acute peritonitis may pass into a condition indicating septic infection.

Symptoms
of septi-
cæmia.

Septicæmia generally sets in between the second and the seventh day, with vomiting, steady rise of temperature, and simultaneous rise of the pulse.

The complexion becomes muddy, the expression dull, a dark-red flush on the cheek, spirits at first depressed, later apathetic.

Condition of tongue and skin varies considerably, as a rule, tongue rough, red, and dry, and skin dry until near death. The tongue may remain moist and skin act profusely throughout.

It is a bad sign when flatus does not pass from the bowel, as is tympanites or distention of the bowels with gas. Another highly unfavorable symptom is persistence of vomiting, especially when the vomited matter is no longer frothy and white, but becomes green or dark.

The treatment of septicæmia is preventive rather than curative. Septicæmia when it has once set in is very unamenable to any kind of treatment. The surgeon sometimes reopens the abdomen and washes it out. The nurse will need to make the preparations for this as nearly as possible like those she made for the original operation. Thorough asepsis should be maintained.

Treatment of septicæmia.

Secondary operation.

For the vomiting, if it be bilious or dark the stomach may have to be washed out. This may be done by means of the stomach pump or a piece of long rubber tubing fitted with a funnel. A weak solution of warm salt water is used for the purpose, being poured in through the funnel, and after sufficient has been introduced into the stomach

Washing out of stomach for vomiting.

to fill it, as will be indicated by the retching of the patient, the funnel may be inverted and placed over a waste pail below the patient, and, the tube acting as a siphon, thus carries off the fluid from the stomach. The introduction of the stomach tube requires no little skill on the part of the nurse. As a rule the surgeon attends to the matter himself. Should the nurse have it to do, she should proceed as follows : first lubricating the outside of the tube with a little glycerine she places the end of it in the patient's mouth and directs her to swallow it. This movement is aided by the nurse holding the tube, and as it enters the œsophagus (or gullet) gently forcing it down the required length. A black ring on the tube, as it approaches the teeth, indicates the point at which the nurse may regard the tube as sufficiently introduced, the ring being on a line with the teeth. The funnel is then connected with the outer end of the tube (if one does not form a part of the apparatus), and the nurse standing at a height on a stool or chair pours in the salt solution slowly at a temperature of from 100°–105° Fahr. The patient will need to be well protected, a rubber cloth being fastened around the neck. In withdrawing the tube it should be done as quickly as possible to prevent retching. Shortly after each washing some liquid nourishment with the addition of stimulants, if necessary, may be given.

Before the vomiting has become so excessive, or before the stomach washing is attempted, it may be found to be of advantage to let the patient sip very hot water containing just a pinch of salt. This measure has been found, as a rule, preferable to the use of bits of ice, especially as it affects the patient afterward in her ability to take food and retain it. *Other measures for control of vomiting.*

The temperature, if over 102°, should be reduced, if possible, by means of the icecap or other apparatus of the kind. After the reduction of temperature and washing out of the stomach, some cases of septicæmia get better, because the poison thrown off by means of the mucous membrane of the stomach is removed by the washing and not reabsorbed into the system. *Reduction of temperature.*

If flatus does not pass freely from the bowel, especially after the insertion of the rectal tube, enemata containing salts, glycerine, turpentine, etc., may be used. Should these prove unsatisfactory, salts may be given by mouth. Because of their depressing effect, it is better to give such in small doses, as one teaspoonful of Rochelle salts dissolved in a tablespoonful of water, once in an hour, until three or four doses are taken. *Enemata for expulsion of flatus.* *Administration of salts, etc., by mouth.*

Doran recommends for the expulsion of flatus one-half teaspoonful of aromatic spirit of ammonia in a little hot water. Beef-tea or milk enemata combined sometimes with stimulants will be needed

10

in addition to what the patient takes by mouth, for the treatment of septicæmia requires the support of the patient's strength for combating the poison.

Saline treat-ment of peritonitis. Where peritonitis alone exists, especial reliance is placed, in this day, upon the saline treatment. An early and thorough evacuation of the bowels, with discharge of flatus, should be obtained. The means employed may be the same as those above mentioned, doses of Rochelle or Epsom salts being administered by mouth, or, if the stomach is not retentive, by rectal enemata.

FIG. 43.

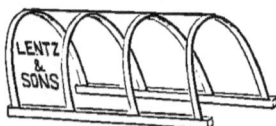

Cradle for Supporting Bedclothes.

Treatment for relief of pain. The pain arising from the tendency to accumulation of gas in the transverse colon and consequent pressure upon the diaphragm may be relieved by the application of warm flaxseed poultices over the lower portion of the chest, renewed once in two hours.

The discomfort caused by the weight of the bed-clothing may be relieved by the use of a bed-cradle.

Bed-cradle. A bed-cradle can be readily improvised by means

of a large barrel-hoop divided in two equal parts. The two semicircles thus produced are then fastened together in the middle with their convexities looking the same way. This forms a coop-like arrangement, which, placed over the patient's body as she lies in bed, supports the bed-clothing quite as well as a more expensive cradle.

Opium is but little used now in the management of peritonitis. The nurse would, however, think of using no remedy, unless the warm poultice, without the direction of the surgeon. The free use of salts has been found to afford speedy relief from pain.

Internal Hemorrhage.—This may come about from a slipping of the ligature, or from vessels which have been severed by the breaking up of adhesions. The danger is greatest in the first day or two, primary hemorrhage occurring, as a rule, within 24 to 48 hours. *Internal hemorrhage.*

Primary hemorrhage.

The symptoms by which the nurse will recognize this condition are faintness, paleness, restlessness, a rapid, thready pulse. The surgeon should at once be sent for. The nurse can do little for this condition, excepting to keep the patient from fainting, by lowering her head and giving her stimulants in small doses, as 1 teaspoonful whisky or brandy in cold water once in 10 to 15 minutes, *Symptoms of hemorrhage.*

Management.

stimulating respiration by inhalation of hartshorn, etc., until the doctor comes. So far as possible the nurse should arrange to have everything in readiness should the doctor suddenly decide to reopen the abdomen. Especially should care be taken to see that a supply of hot sterilized water shall be in readiness.

Intestinal obstruction.

Intestinal Obstruction.—This may occur early or late after an operation. The intestines may from various causes be bent or constricted so as to prevent the passage of their contents beyond a certain point.

This obstruction may cause fatal collapse or even perforation of the intestines.

Symptoms of obstruction.

The symptoms are abdominal pain, constant vomiting, distention of the abdomen, without a marked rise of the temperature.

Prevention.

Much may be done to prevent danger from this source, by proper attention to the bowels before operation.

Methods of relieving.

Change in the position of the patient from one side to another, or inverting the patient by elevating the foot of the bed considerably above the surface, so that the intestines are carried toward the

High injection.

diaphragm ; the use of the high rectal douche, several quarts of water being allowed to flow into the intestines with the patient in an inverted position—any of these methods will sometimes straighten out the bend or loosen the constriction of the intestines.

It has sometimes been found necessary to re-open the abdominal wound and thus to remove the obstruction.

Fæcal Fistula.—This is a small opening in some Fæcal Fistula. part of the intestines which communicates with the abdominal wound, opening on the surface of the body, and permitting the contents of the bowel to pass out at this point. These openings are produced from various causes and are sometimes very slow to close up.

The nurse must exercise the greatest care in changing dressings as often as may be necessary and preventing the contaminating effect of the fæcal matter.

Abscesses.—These may be suture-track abscesses, Abscesses. or may come in the abdominal walls at a point whence the drainage tube was removed, or may be formed by morbid changes in the pedicle. The Symptoms of inflammation in wound. nurse should be quick to report any redness or irritation about the wound, as an abscess may thus be averted. When it once occurs, the abscess should be thoroughly evacuated and the dressings kept properly changed.

Thrombosis.—By this is meant the formation of a Thrombosis. clot in a vein, by which an obstruction to the

circulation is produced.   This causes a swelling of
the limb.   It is not an infrequent result after the
removal of a simple ovarian tumor, particularly if
it be a very large one.   It is generally caused by
the patient's attempting to walk or stand too soon,
as at the end of a fortnight.   In many of these
cases a previous history of swelling of the limb can
Symptoms.: be obtained.   Very frequently the patient simply
complains that one leg feels bigger than the other.
On examination the tissues over the tibia or shin-
bone may seem swollen, but there will be no
especial tenderness.

Phleg-
masia.
Phlegmasia.—By this is meant an inflammation
of the veins caused by a similar obstruction and the
production of inflammation in the walls of the
Symptoms. veins.   The swelling in these cases is generally
marked and extends to the thigh; enlarged, tender,
cord-like veins may be felt in the groin, or under
the knee, or elsewhere.   There is apt to be considerable constitutional disturbance, fever, and
severe pain.

Manage-
ment of
thrombosis
and phleg-
masia.
Whenever any sign of thrombosis occurs the
patient should be kept in the recumbent position.
The swollen limb should be kept warm by the
application around it of cotton or wool.   Over the
swollen cord-like veins a warm flaxseed poultice may be placed for the relief of pain.   The
application on lint, beneath this poultice, of an oint-

ment, made by combining equal parts of belladonna and iodine ointment, will often serve to allay more quickly the swelling and pain. The limb should be elevated by pillows or a fracture box, forming an inclined plane. The bowels should receive careful attention, free purgation being obtained by any means the surgeon may prescribe. It is of extreme importance to keep the limb still, even after the swelling has subsided. The patient must not be permitted to place her foot on the ground until the surgeon gives his full consent, for this complication is a most serious one, and is a cause for anxiety.

Pulmonary Embolism.—This is a fatal complica- Embolism. tion produced by a small clot being swept through the current of the circulation into the pulmonary artery, forming thus an obstruction to the circulation and producing instant death. Young, active patients, whom it is difficult to keep sufficiently quiet after an operation, are especially in danger from this cause.

Cases have been reported where patients died suddenly from this complication days and even weeks after an operation, when all appeared to be going on well. It may occur, as a result of over- Complications. exertion, in any disease accompanied by debility or exhaustion.

Parotitis.—Inflammation of the parotid glands, Parotitis.

such as occurs in mumps, is sometimes found as a complication after abdominal section. In some cases this is simply a temporary swelling which disappears in a few days; in others it may be septic in character, when suppuration may result, or even inflammation of the periosteum and destruction of the lower jaw. The management, if septic, will be that of septicæmia—supporting in character. Such local applications for relief of pain, etc., must be employed as are ordered by the surgeon.

Palpitation.

Palpitation.—Severe attacks of palpitation are apt to occur after abdominal section, and most frequently occur at night. It is supposed that these

Causes.

are caused by changes in the circulation, due to removal of a tumor, and, possibly, in large part to enforced lying on the back for considerable length

Management.

of time. A half teaspoonful of aromatic spirit of ammonia in two tablespoonfuls of water will give the patient great relief. The symptom may greatly alarm an inexperienced nurse, but any expression of fright on her part only makes the patient worse, hence she should not allow her anxiety to be seen. The condition is not a dangerous one.

Cystitis.

Cystitis.—Inflammation of the bladder quite frequently occurs as a complication after abdominal

Symptoms.

section. The patient complains of pain in the lower part of the abdomen, and feels cutting pains on passing her urine. Sometimes the irritation

shows itself simply in a frequent desire to pass
water. The urine is generally thick with ropy
mucus and contains a considerable amount of sediment. The difficulty of passing water in urinals or Causes.
bedpans in the recumbent posture is partly
responsible for this. The more frequent cause is
improper catheterism. The awkward use of the
catheter, which leads a nurse to carry discharges
from the vagina into the urethra and bladder; or
the use of a catheter which is not aseptic, not having been kept properly cleansed, are prominent
causes for such trouble. The free use of flaxseed Management.
tea or barley water, with a stoppage of the use of
the catheter, will often be sufficient to put a stop to
the suffering. The use of medicinal remedies in
case of too great acidity or alkalinity of the urine
will have to be directed by the surgeon. The nurse Testing of
urine.
should have a little litmus paper, which can readily
be obtained at any apothecary's, and test the urine,
so that she can report its reaction to the surgeon.
If the blue litmus paper is turned a decided red
when dipped in the urine, the secretion is too
acid; if the pink litmus be turned blue we have
an alkaline urine.

It is sometimes necessary, for the comfort of the Washing
out of
patient, to wash out the bladder with some soothing bladder.
solution, as a saturated solution of boric acid. The
apparatus necessary for this is simply a soft rubber

Nelaton catheter, a small funnel which can slip into its outer end, and a small pitcher containing the solution to be used in the process. The solution should range in temperature from 100°–105° Fahr., not higher. The patient being placed on the pan, the urine contained in the bladder is first entirely drawn off by means of the catheter; its outer extremity is then elevated, the funnel fitted in and the solution gently allowed to flow into the bladder until the patient experiences a sense of distention of the bladder; the funnel may then be inverted over the bedpan, and the liquid allowed to flow out. This cleanses the bladder of all debris. It may then be refilled to distention, and again emptied so long as the liquid does not come away clear. After the liquid becomes clear, the bladder may be refilled with the solution and the catheter withdrawn, allowing the solution to remain in the bladder for its medicinal effect upon the inflamed mucous membrane. The patient will probably retain this some little time before passing it.

Return catheter.

The return or double-channel catheter is sometimes used in preference to the apparatus just described, but in my opinion is not so convenient. The nurse should never attempt washing out the bladder without the surgeon's instruction and sanction.

Occasionally the nurse is directed to place warm

flaxseed poultices over the lower part of the abdo- Poultices
men for the relief of the bladder irritation. This pain.
cannot always be resorted to, because of the close
proximity of the wound to the part. Should the
poultices be ordered, the nurse should see that
they are changed with sufficient frequency to keep
them warm, as they are worse than useless when
cold. A poultice of ordinary size, if well covered
with oiled silk and a layer of cotton or wool, will
retain its warmth about two hours.

Tetanus.—This is a disease which consists in a Tetanus.
permanent contraction of all or some of the muscles.
Its characteristics are closure of the jaws, difficulty
or impossibility of swallowing, rigidity of the limbs
and trunk. The trunk is sometimes curved forward (emprosthotonus), sometimes backward (opis-
thotonus), and sometimes to one side (pleurotho-
tonus).

When tetanus is confined to the muscles of the Trismus.
jaws it is called trismus.

It is a most formidable condition. This disease,
although rare after abdominal section, may occur,
as after other operations.

Treatment is of little avail. It must be treated Treatment.
here as where it complicates other diseases, that is
by blood-letting, cold and warm bathing, anæsthe-
tics, opiates, etc., according to the surgeon's direc-

tion. The nurse's duty is to report the first indications of such an occurrence.

The surgeon may desire to reopen the abdomen for examination of the stump for any special source of irritation.

Passage of ligatures.

Passage of Ligatures.—When the pedicle of the tumor suppurates, the ligatures may be discharged through the bladder, or through the bowels, or through an abscess of the abdominal wall. This may occur at varying lengths of time after the operation.

Menstruation after abdominal section.

Menstruation after Abdominal Section.—A "show" of blood frequently occurs a few days after operation, particularly after ovariotomy or operation upon the uterine appendages. There is almost always some rise in temperature accompanying this "show" and frequently depression of spirits. The pulse, too, may rise considerably.

Necessity for rest.

The patient must always be advised to keep very quiet during the first three or four periods after an abdominal section, particularly for disease of the pelvic organs, as there may be hemorrhage from the stump.

CHAPTER XIII.

THE PELVIC ORGANS IN WOMEN.

These are divided into the external and internal organs of generation. The external organs are also called the "pudenda" or "vulva." External and internal genitalia.

Immediately above the pubic bone, or anterior border of the pelvis, is a cushion of fat, usually covered with hair. This is called the "mons veneris." — Mons veneris.

On each side of the opening of the vulva are the labia majora, or large lips. Lying beneath these and concealed by them in young women, are two thin folds of flesh, named the "labia minora" or "nymphæ." They join together above, and at their junction is a small projecting body called the "clitoris." — Labia majora. Nymphæ. Clitoris.

The small triangular space between the clitoris and the nymphæ is the vestibule. — Vestibule.

The opening of the urethra (the "meatus urinarius"), through which the urine escapes from the bladder, is in the middle of the lower border of the vestibule. — Meatus urinarius.

It is very important that the nurse should know

157

the exact position of the meatus urinarius, as she will frequently be called upon to pass the catheter.

Vaginal orifice.

Below the vestibule is the orifice of the vagina,

FIG. 44.

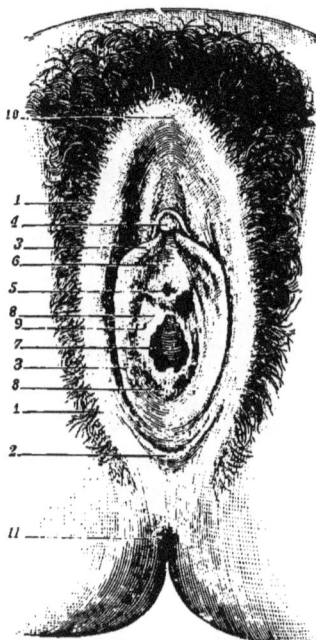

1. The right large lip. 2. The fourchette. 3. Right nympha. 4. Clitoris. 5. Urethral orifice. 6. Vestibule. 7. Orifice of vagina. 8. Hymen. 10. Mons veneris. 11. Anal orifice.

the canal leading to the uterus or womb. In virgins a delicate membrane, usually crescentic in shape, blocks the entrance to the vagina.

The hymen is usually ruptured at marriage, but Hymen.
a woman may be a virgin, yet have no hymen.
In some cases it persists even after marriage and
offers an obstruction at childbirth. A woman who
has borne children has a few fleshy projections at
the orifice of the vagina, the only remains of the
hymen, called the "carunculæ myrtiformes." Be- Carunculæ myrti- formes.
tween the vulva and the anus is a mass of flesh,
the space on the surface measuring 1½ inches in
length. During the birth of the child this becomes
greatly distended, and thins like rubber. This is Perineum.
the perineum. It may be torn during labor to a
greater or less extent; sometimes it is completely
torn into the bowel.

That part of the perineum in the virgin which
forms the posterior border of the vulva, is called
the "fourchette." It is merely a fold of skin, and Fourchette.
is almost always torn in a first labor.

Behind the perineum is the anus, or orifice of Anal ori- fice.
the rectum—the lower part of the bowel.

The vagina is a canal connecting the external Vagina.
with the internal organs of generation.

The uterus is at the top of the vagina. In front Uterus.
of the uterus is the bladder, and behind and to the
left, the rectum.

A secretion of mucus keeps the vagina moist.
There should, however, be no discharge in a perfectly healthy woman. During pregnancy, and as

a result of ill-health or local inflammation, the natural secretion may be greatly increased, and the patient is then said to have " the whites."

In labor the discharge is very greatly increased, so as to aid the birth of the child.

The uterus is a pear-shaped organ, 3 inches in length, 1 ½ inches in breadth, and about 1 inch in

FIG. 45.

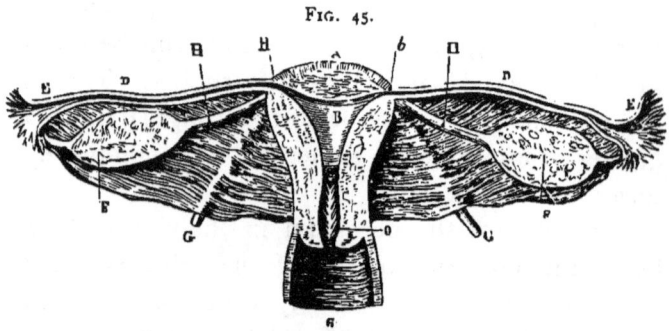

Cavity of the Uterus and Fallopian Tubes.

A. Superior border or fundus of the womb. *B.* Cavity of the womb. *C.* Cavity of the neck of the womb. *D.* Canal of the Fallopian tube. *E.* The fimbriated extremity. *F, F.* The ovaries. *G.* The cavity of the vagina.

thickness. It weighs a little over an ounce in its normal condition in a virgin. After child-bearing it remains larger and heavier than before. That portion of the uterus which communicates with the Cervix.   vagina is called the neck, or *cervix*. The chief portion of the organ above this is called the *body*, and

the rounded upper surface the *fundus*. The opening in the cervix which communicates with the vagina is called the "os uteri." That portion of the   Os uteri.
cervix in front of the os uteri is the anterior lip,
while that part which lies behind is the posterior
lip.

The Fallopian tubes are two canals which pass   Fallopian tubes.
from each side of the upper portion of the uterus.
They are from 3 to 4½ inches long and will admit
the passage of a bristle.

Each ends in a trumpet-shaped opening sur-
rounded by a fringe of small projections called
"fimbriæ." This is called the fimbriated extremity.   Fimbriated extremity.
When the ovum (or egg) escapes from the ovary,
it is received by the Fallopian tube and reaches the
cavity of the uterus in this way.

The ovaries are two small flattened bodies about   Ovaries.
an inch long and half an inch thick. They lie
about an inch from the fundus of the uterus on
each side, in the folds of the broad ligament. The   Broad ligaments.
broad ligaments are folds of peritoneum, a thin
glistening membrane which covers the uterus and
all the pelvic organs, and by means of which the
uterus is suspended in the pelvis. The bladder
and rectum being covered with the same tissue,
there is an intimate connection between the three,
so that if one is deranged the others are likely to
be so also.

Breasts.   The breasts are considered as belonging to the external organs of generation. They are two glands situated on the front of the chest, one on each side of the breast-bone. They vary in size and shape in different women, and during pregnancy they enlarge greatly.

They secrete milk for the nourishment of the child. The nipple at the apex of the gland is a conical-shaped projection. The milk ducts all come towards it from the different parts of the breast and open on its surface. The areola is a pink or brown circle which surrounds the nipple.

There is an intimate connection between the breasts and the uterus. Pain in the breast may be the result of disease of the uterus. The secretion of milk is called " *lactation.*"

Menstruation.   Menstruation is a bloody discharge from the uterus every month. It begins usually about the age of fourteen and recurs every month except during pregnancy or while a woman is nursing. It ceases at the change of life or menopause (between forty-five and fifty).

Puberty.   At *puberty,* that is when this function first appears, the girl becomes a woman, the breasts enlarge and the pelvis increases in size. The organs of generation become ready to perform the functions of reproduction.

The menstrual flow recurs every twenty-eight

days and lasts about four days. The quantity of blood lost at a period is from four to eight ounces. Different women vary much in this respect. The discharge is blood mixed with mucus. Its color is dark red. Any peculiarity in color or the appearance of any clots in the discharge will need to be noticed by the nurse, and the discharge kept for the doctor's inspection. There is usually a feeling of discomfort at the menstrual period, with headache, pains in the back, breasts, etc. These symptoms are more severe in some women than in others.

Periodicity of menstrual flow.

Quantity of menstrual flow.

Accompanying symptoms.

Conception most usually takes place immediately or very soon after a period. This is not an invariable rule, as women have become pregnant before menstruation has been established or even after the menopause. They may also become pregnant while nursing.

Conception.

A nurse is so often questioned on these points that it is well for her to have information concerning them. Always endeavoring to discourage the inquisitiveness of mere prurient curiosity, she should aim to give wise counsel concerning matters of which her patient may hesitate to speak to her physician. In doing so, the nurse should, however, speak to the physician of any matters of importance concerning the condition of the patient, which she may thus learn, and ask his counsel as to the advice she should give.

CHAPTER XIV.

DISEASES OF WOMEN.

Definition.   By this term is meant, in particular, the diseases affecting the organs peculiar to women, as the external and internal genitals. The term may be made to include diseases of the rectum and bladder, which are closely associated with these organs, and also diseases of the breasts.

Causes of disease.   In investigating the causes of pelvic disease, we find that ignorance on the part of women. is largely responsible for their great number and frequency of occurrence. Civilization, so called, has laid certain restrictions on healthful living and established fashions which are directly opposed to physiological laws, and which tend to produce abnormal conditions.

Some of the most common causes of pelvic diseases are—

1. Neglect of physical exercise, especially in the open air.

2. Improper clothing.

3. Improper and insufficient food.   .

164

4. Habitual neglect of the functions of the bowels and bladder.

5. Imprudence during menstruation.

6. Overstrain of the nervous system by too much excitement, unwholesome reading, unwholesome companions, unwholesome thought.

7. Marriage when disease of the genital organs exists.

8. Lack of prudence in the marital relations.

9. Prevention of conception.

10. Induction of abortion.

11. Neglect of injuries due to parturition or childbirth.

Within recent years it has become more customary for women to take physical exercise : girls may play tennis, row, ride on horseback, and take long walks, without being regarded as unlady-like. *Lack of physical exercise, sunlight, and fresh air.*

Even yet, however, so much of woman's work lies within the walls of her home that she is apt to become careless on this point, to lose all taste for out-door exercise and to confine herself to heated, illy-ventilated rooms. For amusement she takes up reading, music, drawing, or some other light task, which keeps her sitting, so that her muscular system becomes weakened. It is not only bodily exertion, however, that she needs, but the exhilarating effect of sunlight and fresh air—the mental relaxation which comes from out-door exercise.

Every healthy woman should walk at least two miles daily and observe the manner of walking which will serve to exercise her muscles to their fullest extent and thus stimulate the circulation—a brisk walk with the head held erect and the shoulders thrown well back, so that the lungs may, at the same time, be well filled with air. So important is it to keep the general circulation in good condition that in the management of conditions of local congestion or inflammation which interfere with active exercise, the use of passive motion by the Swedish movement cure, massage, Turkish baths, or frequent salt baths combined with calisthenics are much resorted to in treatment.

Improper clothing.

In the style of clothing worn by women the last few years have made a great change. It is no longer necessary for a woman to dress injuriously to health in order to be well dressed. The patterns of the Jenness-Miller Reform Dress Wear and other dress reform systems aim to correct former unhygienic requirements. The constriction of the chest caused by the use of corsets; pressure and partial paralysis of the abdominal and chest muscles by tight and heavy clothing; the unnatural position of the pelvic organs as a result of such pressure, were the inevitable result of former fashionable modes of dressing. To a certain extent these deleterious styles still prevail, and women who are ignorant of physiological laws, by adopting such fashions keep them up. Intelligent women who desire to live long and happily, and to provide a future of physical comfort for their children, are ready to adopt the reform systems which correct these errors.

The clothing should all be supported from the shoulders, and should be so constructed as to

Hygienic dressing.

Fig. 46.

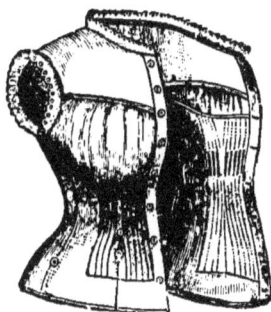

Equipoise Waist.

allow perfect freedom of every part of the body. The use of the Jenness-Miller model bodice or Equipoise waist—to which the skirts and undergarments may all be fastened, is an excellent method of attaining this purpose. The jersey-fitting union undergarment of silk or merino may be worn in addition, if desired. Divided skirts or leglettes made of muslin or, in winter, of flannel, cashmere, or silk, etc., make a very comfortable undergarment and enable one to dispense with underskirts. The skirts of dresses may be fastened, by means of buttonholes in the waistband, to the Equipoise waist or model bodice. If heavy, however, it is best to have them fastened to a separate waist, modeled after the pattern of the child's petticoat waist with armholes. Were these methods more strictly observed in the dressing of growing girls, fewer women would be found suffering from displacements of the uterus and ovaries and the many pelvic diseases which follow in their wake.

Improper and insufficient food.   Poor blood as a result of poor eating is so common an accompaniment of uterine disease that we must often regard it as the chief cause of the abnormal condition. The muscular tone of the pelvic organs is decidedly affected by want of sufficient nutrient material, and displacements are thus readily produced. It is not only important that a certain amount of food shall be taken daily, but the food should be such as is capable of making blood of good quality. It should be nourishing and digestible. Pastry and sweets should be avoided or taken only in small amount. The meals should be so regulated that a heavy meal shall not be taken at night when the digestive processes are least active. Milk, eggs, meat, bread, fresh vegetables and fruit should be properly combined in forming a whole-some dietary.

Habitual constipation and lack of attention to the bladder are frequent causes of uterine displace-ment. The uterus lying, as it does, between the bladder and bowel is readily affected by the condi-tion of either. Not realizing this, women are often led, from motives of modesty, to neglect attending to their demands, and thus they acquire a habit of toleration which is most injurious. The large hard masses of fecal matter which remain not only for days, but often for a week at a time in the rectum, interfere with the circulation in the pelvic organs, and produce displacements which are sometimes most unmanageable, in fact, incurable. A full bladder acts similarly by pressure on the anterior surface of the uterus, and, in addition, the retention of urine may become a source of disease both of the bladder and of the kidneys. *Habitual neglect of the functions of bowels and bladder.*

Violent or excessive physical exercise is to be avoided during menstruation, because of the con-gested condition of the pelvic organs at this time. For the same reason precaution should be taken regarding undue exposure to cold, or sudden chill-ing from imprudence in bathing. The suppression which is often thus induced is a result of over-congestion and a direct cause of uterine and ovarian disease. Excessive emotion frequently produces *Imprudence during menstrua-tion.*

similar results. Hence scenes of excitement should be avoided at such times. Exposure due to insufficient clothing, the low neck and bare arms of fashionable evening dress, have frequently been the cause of life-long ill health.

Nervous overstrain.   Tension upon the nervous system is partly the result of our fast modes of living—the competition of the day which makes each one strive to surpass his neighbor. It is also largely the result of inheritance, education, and habit. This unfortunate combination of circumstances offers a formidable resistance to one's efforts to gain self-control. Determination and continued effort, however, accomplish much in the formation of habits which give one a capacity for endurance. The diversion of the mind into wholesome trains of thought and study will serve to hold in abeyance the impulses of one's nature. Sources of excitement, such as persistent novel-reading, a frequenting of places of amusement, extreme indulgence in society gatherings, are to be avoided.

One of the greatest difficulties a nurse will meet will be the management of a mind thus diseased, and infinite tact and skill will be necessary to enable her to steer the thoughts and purposes of her patient into safe channels. The nurse must make the moral atmosphere of the sick-room.

Marriage.   Marriage when disease of the genital organs

exists is another frequent source of disease. The reason for this may clearly be seen. Organs already the seat of a morbid process are only more extensively irritated by the increased congestion thus induced.

Lack of prudence in the marital relations in a Lack of prudence. similar way may cause disease. Periods during which the pelvic organs are in a state of congestion from natural or abnormal causes, should be periods of rest. Thus during the menstrual period and for a short time before and after the same, during pregnancy and the lying-in, the pelvic organs demand rest.

Prevention of conception and induction of abor- Prevention of conception. tion act in the same way as the last two causes mentioned, that is, they result in conditions of excessive congestion and even active inflammation which not only bring about diseased conditions which cause much suffering, but which endanger the life of the patient. Blood-poisoning is not an uncommon result of efforts at inducing abortion.

Neglect of injuries due to childbirth is a most Induction of abortion common cause of disease. Lacerations, erosions, Injuries due to etc., frequently pass unnoticed by the physician. child-birth. The nurse in cleansing her patient after delivery, has an opportunity to observe them, and should be careful to call the attention of the physician to their existence. This should always be done elsewhere

than in the presence of the patient.	The best time
to repair these injuries is as soon as possible after
their occurrence.	Should their repair for various
reasons be put off for a time, they should not be
forgotten, but the advice of a competent physician obtained as to the probability of their inducing
chronic forms of pelvic disease.

CHAPTER XV.

GENERAL NURSING IN PELVIC DISEASES.

From what has been said in the preceding chapter it will be seen that it is seldom that a nurse will be called upon to take charge of a case of pelvic trouble, that she will not find the patient suffering from many morbid conditions. She will have poor blood, poor circulation, poor appetite, poor digestion, poor nerves. She will suffer from cold hands and feet, indigestion, constipation, headache, backache, sleeplessness, and extreme nervousness. The nurse will have abundant opportunity to exercise all that ingenuity and skill can devise to meet this array of ills. *Symptoms of pelvic disease.*

The physician's directions will include—

1. Attention to diet.
2. Stimulation of the circulation and respiration by bathing, exercise, etc. *Management.*
3. Regulation of the sleep.
4. Regulation of the functions of the body.
5. Regulation of the clothing.
6. Treatment of local conditions of disease.
7. Mental occupation.

173

Forced
feeding.

The patient will probably be placed upon " forced feeding ; " that is, she will be made to take a certain amount of nourishment in the twenty-four hours. The food will be prescribed by the physician according to the especial requirements in each case. The milk diet is frequently used where digestion and assimilation are poor. Beef-tea is sometimes used, alternating with milk ; a gill or a gill and a half of each may be given once in two hours. It may be necessary to have these peptonized. Should the liquid milk diet tend to produce flatus it may be of advantage to thicken the milk with rice flour, wheat flour, crumbed bread, etc. ; junket, or milk thickened with rennet, is often liked by many patients, and is easily digested ; farina, wheat germ, egg custard, and similar preparations, if well prepared, may be quite readily digested and help to vary the monotony. The chief objection to the milk diet arises from its monotony ; the patient gets to dislike it, so that it is almost impossible to get her to take sufficient nourishment. By a little management the nurse can put off this period. A drop of black coffee, or extract of vanilla in a glass of milk, or a little salt, will so change the flavor as to make it more palatable. The addition of lime water, a tablespoonful or two to a glass of milk (1 ½ gills) is sometimes necessary to aid the digestion.

Milk diet.

Where the patient does not need to be kept on liquid food, or when the dietary can be increased, fresh animal food can be given three times a day, and as much other nutritious food as the patient can take—stale bread, rice, eggs, crushed wheat, etc. Between breakfast and dinner, dinner and supper, and on retiring at night, the patient should take a tumblerful of milk or a cup of beef-tea, or of beef, mutton, or chicken broth. *Mixed diet.*

Should the patient be entirely on liquid diet she should receive nourishment about once in three hours through the night. *Night feeding.*

A very anæmic patient may need to be fed once or twice through the night, even when taking a mixed diet.

Where meats are not well digested, it has been found, in our experience, that the raw-beef sandwich, made by scraping a tender piece of raw beefsteak with a knife, salting and spreading the pulp thus obtained between thin slices of bread or toast, offers a convenient and palatable form of administering animal food. Beef being the most nutritious of the animal foods, a tender piece of broiled beefsteak, or a slice or two of rare roastbeef, or the raw-beef sandwich, should frequently form a part of the meal. All fried foods, pastry, and sweet desserts should be avoided. When the stomach is very irritable, and only small quantities of food can *Animal food.*

be taken, freshly expressed beef-juice gives a highly concentrated and nutritious food, 1 tablespoonful of this representing the nutritive properties of about one-quarter of a pound of beef.

Bathing.—A sponge bath of warm water strongly impregnated with salt should be taken each morning on rising, and, if possible, at night on retiring. A teacupful of ordinary table salt may be added to **Stimulation of skin.** the basin of warm water. Rocksalt may be obtained for bathing purposes, and kept on hand if preferred. This sponging should be followed by a brisk rubbing with a coarse towel; the knitted tape-towel is the best, or a bathing glove of coarse material, or a flesh brush may be used.

Calisthenic exercises with dumb-bells, rods, etc., **Exercise.** or the practice of Swedish movements from ten to fifteen minutes following each bath, are of great value.

Any active exercise to be taken by the patient must be controlled by the physician. If the patient is unable to take such, the use of massage and tonic electricity will be called into play. A good nurse should understand the methods of applying both massage and electricity for their **Rules for exercise.** tonic effect. Neither should be given within two hours of a full meal, either before or after. Neither should be given when the patient is very tired, nor should the application be made to exhaustion. An hour's massage is the average length of time for a patient who has learned to take it without growing tired. The application of electricity, that is by Electricity. means of the faradic battery, will require from twenty minutes to half an hour for the entire body. The patient should be kept well protected from exposure during these applications.

A patient who is entirely dependent upon passive exercise and who is not too weak, may have one of these applications in the morning and the other in the afternoon or at bedtime. When the patient suffers from sleeplessness, the massage given at Massage. bedtime has often a most calming and healthful effect, serving to induce sleep. In any case, at whatever time of day these applications may be given, the patient should remain quietly at rest in bed for a half an hour to an hour after the treatment, and if possible take a nap.

Sleep.—A patient in this generally run-down Sleep. condition demands a great deal of sleep, and should try to obtain at least nine hours every night, beside the hour in the daytime. The habit of retiring early should be cultivated, as sleep is far more refreshing when thus taken in the early hours of the night. The patient should be asleep at least by nine o'clock. She will then be prepared for early rising and the enjoyment of the hours of the day which are most invigorating.

12

Clothing.—Something of what is required in this connection has already been stated in the preceding chapter. The clothing should be loose, light, and supported from the shoulders. It should also be sufficiently warm to aid in keeping up the warmth of the surface of the body. Sudden changes in the atmosphere should be provided for, and additional clothing employed to protect from chilling.

Rules regarding clothing.

Remedies prescribed by the physician should be carefully given and their effect upon the functions of the body observed and noted. The bowels should be thoroughly evacuated once in twenty-four hours. If this is not a free movement, or if its passage is attended with difficulty, bringing about straining, the matter should be reported. The use of some saline water, as Hunyadi Janos, a half tumblerful once or twice daily, and the proper use of massage over the abdomen in the daily treatment may bring about a permanent cure of this trouble. The color and consistency of the movements should be likewise observed.

Function of bowels.

The quantity of urine passed in twenty-four hours should be noted. The usual amount in health is between forty and fifty fluid ounces. It may rise as high as eighty fluid ounces. The variation depends greatly upon the amount of fluid taken. The urine may be scanty when the patient has abstained from liquids, or when water

Function of kidneys.

has been eliminated in excess by skin or bowels. Thus free sweats or a persistent diarrhœa will greatly affect the quantity of urine passed in one day. Any diminution of the urine which approaches suppression is of grave import and should be promptly reported. Temporary excess in the flow of urine will occur after hysterical paroxysms and other convulsive attacks. The color, quantity, reaction, and presence or absence of sediment should be noted.

Any disturbance of the digestion must be carefully reported to the physician, as it is exceedingly important that digestion and assimilation should do their part to restore the broken-down system. *Disturbance of digestion.*

Vaginal Injections.—The treatment of conditions of disease of the pelvic organs very frequently calls for the use of vaginal injections.

Various methods have been suggested for giving these, and several different forms of vaginal syringe have been invented. The Davidson hand-ball syringe, or the Davidson fountain syringe, are those probably most frequently employed. The method as described by Emmett, who was the first gynæcologist in this country to employ such douches extensively in his practice, is as follows :— *Methods of giving vaginal injections.*

" The injection can be better given to the patient after she is undressed for the night, and in bed. She should be placed near the edge of the bed, with the hips elevated as much as possible by the bedpan, and a small pillow under her back, the lower limbs being flexed.

" Her body must be covered, to protect her from cold and her position made perfectly comfortable; whenever the bed is a soft one, for the purpose of keeping the hips elevated a broad board should be

FIG. 47.

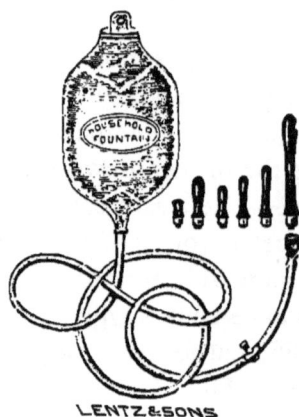

Fountain Syringe.

placed under the pan to prevent it from sinking into the bed from the weight of the patient. The vessel of hot water is placed on a chair by the bedside, and the nurse passes the nozzle of the syringe into the vagina, over the perineum, directing it along the recto-vaginal wall (that is, the posterior wall of the vagina), until it reaches the posterior cul-de-sac (the portion of the vagina back of the neck of the womb).

"The water must be thrown in at first very carefully, until the vagina has become distended."

In place of the interrupted stream used by working the hand-ball syringe, as described in this method, the fountain syringe, the reservoir of which should be hung several feet above the patient's head, may be employed to even greater advantage, as it permits a continuous stream to flow into the vagina, and does away with the danger of the introduction of air or the forcible injection of water into the uterine cavity in cases where the uterine os has been torn.

In private practice and in the absence of a nurse, the patient is often dependent upon herself for this treatment, hence she should be taught how to arrange for this.   Dr. T. G. Thomas, of New York, suggests the following plan :   "The patient places a pillow upon the edge of her bed, and an empty tub upon the floor under it.   She then covers the pillow by a piece of india-rubber cloth which drapes into the tub.   Then putting two chairs, one on each side and a little in front of the tub, she places a small table in front of these, and upon this another chair.   Upon the chair which stands on the table a tub containing about two gallons of hot water is now put, near the bottom of which has been inserted a spigot to which a long rubber tube is affixed, which ends in a vaginal nozzle. The patient now lies upon the bed, the pelvis elevated by the pillow, places her feet upon the chairs, covers her limbs with a shawl or blanket, touches the spring—an ordinary clothes-pin makes a good one —which controls the flow, and the water bathes the vagina and running out is conducted by the india-rubber cloth into the tub. Here the only articles purchased are the tub with the spigot and tube attached, and a yard of india-rubber cloth, which are inexpensive."

Special apparatus.

In our own practice in the hospital wards we are accustomed to using, as a reservoir for the water, a large copper kettle which holds several gallons of water, called the douche-can. A spigot with rubber tubing is attached to the lower part of this. A rubber bedpan with inflated border and outlet tubing, as shown in the cut, is employed, being placed on the edge of the bed upon a board, if the bed be yielding. It is well to protect the bedding beneath by means of a piece of rubber cloth. This may be long enough to drape down over the edge of the bed and be spread out upon the floor, the waste bucket being placed on it. The patient lies with the bedpan adjusted under her, a pillow placed beneath her back to give it support. The

douche-can filled with hot water, to which any
medicinal agent may be added, as directed by the
physician, is placed upon a high stand, or on a
stool or box placed on a table at the head of the
patient's bed; the spigot being turned and the vaginal nozzle attached to the tubing properly adjusted, the water flows into the vagina and thence
into the rubber pan.   Overflow is prevented by the

FIG. 48.

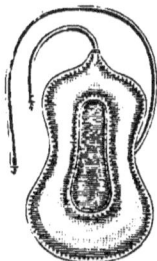

LENTZ&SONS

Rubber Bedpan.

water emptying into the waste bucket through the
outlet tubing.

A form of syringe, which enables the patient to
do without a bedpan, has recently been devised.
It is known as the Gordon Utero-Vaginal Irrigator. . The nozzle is adjusted near a bulb, which is
intended to fit into the vaginal orifice, and thus obstruct the return flow from the vulva.   An outlet
of metal is connected with this bulb, and to it a

long piece of rubber tubing is attached, which communicates with a waste bucket. The patient lies,
as before described, on the edge of the bed, with
her limbs drawn up, a piece of rubber cloth beneath
her hips. The reservoir containing the water to be
used is placed at the head of the bed, elevated some

FIG. 49.

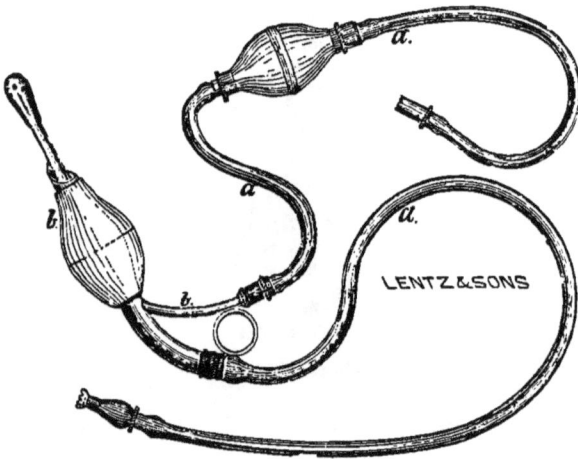

Utero-Vaginal Irrigator.

distance above the level on which the patient lies.
The tubing from the reservoir is connected with the
receiving pipe of the bulb. Through this the water
passes into the vagina, and is carried away by the
outlet pipe and tubing. The bulb should be air-

tight, for unless fully distended the water will escape through the vulva from around it and the
value of the apparatus will be destroyed. The size
of the bulb will of necessity have to correspond to
the size of the vulva. This syringe, when it works
well, is not only of advantage as doing away with
the bedpan, but will enable the douche to be taken
at a much higher temperature than ordinary, for
the water does not flow over the skin on its exit
from the vulva, which is far more susceptible to the
effect of heat than is mucous membrane. A tem-

FIG. 50.

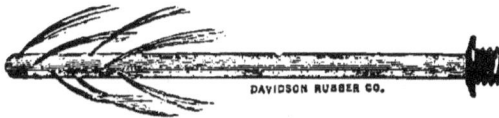

DAVIDSON RUBBER CO.

Vaginal Nozzle with Reverse Current.

perature of from 120°–125° Fahr. can thus readily be borne. The nozzle of a vaginal syringe
should have no opening at its extremity, but should
be made so that a reverse rather than a direct current may be obtained.

Where vaginal injections are intended for medi- Position in
cinal effect it is best that they should be taken which vaginal injec-
lying down. In no other way can the water be tions are
taken.
carried so effectually to the diseased parts. When
required only for cleanliness they may be adminis-

tered in the upright posture, the patient being seated over a vessel. A convenient method is that of placing in a tub the water to be used—one or two gallons. The patient may seat herself over this on a board placed across it, or upon a stool placed in it, and inject the water by means of a hand-ball syringe. The long nozzle being used, the water may be thus made to bathe the cervix. When pessaries are worn, a daily cleansing injection is essential.

The tampon.

The Tampon.—Many pelvic maladies are treated by the use of the tampon, or pledget of cotton or wool saturated or anointed with some medicinal agent. These may be placed by the physician daily, or two or three times weekly. It will be the nurse's duty to have these tampons in readiness. They may be made by cutting strips in the length of a lap of cotton or wool, from six to eight inches long, doubling these strips and tying a piece of twine about six inches in length to one extremity.

Preparation for use of tampon.

Before the tampons are placed the vagina should be cleansed by an antiseptic injection, as bichloride of mercury 1–4000. As the medicinal applications used have frequently the effect of increasing the mucous discharge from the vagina, a napkin should be worn after these treatments. The cotton should be removed, at the time appointed by the physician, by drawing upon the string. It should be wrapped in a piece of paper and burned, or thrown down a privy vault—never in a water-closet, as it will cause stoppage of the waste pipes. The patient should then receive a thorough vaginal injection.

Pessaries.—Should the patient have a pessary adjusted, that is a support for the displaced uterus, the nurse should not permit her to move about if it caused her pain, at least until the physician acquiesced in her doing so. Any unusual complaint of pain or increase of vaginal discharge from its pressure, should be reported to the physician. A patient should understand fully that it is unsafe to wear such a support without the supervision of a physician, who shall advise her as to the necessity of having it removed from time to time for cleansing and replacement or entire removal.

Counter-irritation over the lower part of the abdomen may occasionally be called for in the form of blisters, ointments, poultices, etc. In the management of these the nurse should follow the ordinary rules for their application elsewhere. Poultices of flaxseed, or hot-packs, should, if required for warmth, be applied frequently enough to keep up warmth, about once in two hours. The latter consist of pieces of flannel or several layers of soft muslin wrung out of boiling water, to which a little glycerine may or may not be added. These

Pessaries.

Counter-irritation.

are applied as a poultice, being covered by a piece of oiled silk or muslin, and to still more effectually prevent evaporation, by a layer of cotton wool. An abdominal binder, held in place by a perineal bandage or an ordinary T-bandage, will serve to keep these applications in place. Ointments are best applied on patent lint or soft Canton flannel. They should be spread the thickness of a knife-blade. The best means of keeping such applications in place is by strips of rubber adhesive plaster. A piece of oiled silk or cotton batting should be applied over this to prevent the greasing of the clothing.

Blisters.   A blister should be carefully watched and removed as soon as the scarf-skin fills up with liquid beneath it. If it seems slow in rising, as it should in five to six hours, a flaxseed poultice applied over it will hasten the process. In dressing the blister, care should be taken not to remove the scarf-skin, but clipping a small opening in the most dependent part of the blister, the liquid may be soaked up by absorbent cotton or soft rags, and the blistered surface dressed with cold cream, cosmoline, etc., applied on lint. The fluid from the blister should not be allowed to run over the skin elsewhere, as it will produce irritation.

Mental occupation.   *Mental Occupation.*—The more entirely a nervous patient's mind can be kept occupied with other

things than herself, the more successfully may she
be treated. Upon the nurse will devolve the duty
of supplying wholesome for unwholesome thoughts.
For this reason, if none other, a nurse should keep
up as far as possible, a knowledge of the events of
the day. She should be able to talk to her patient
about the world and its doings, and thus help to
widen her horizon and prevent the fret and worry
which result from a persistent contemplation of
small woes. All gossip should be carefully avoided.
It is necessary that the nurse should be a good
reader, and should train herself to read aloud, for
she may in this way while away many a weary hour
which might otherwise be spent in profitless
thought. As additional recreation for younger
patients particularly are some of the card games,
or puzzles, etc., which are interesting because of
the incentive they give to thought.

With infinite tact a patient may be thus led, Value of tact.
without knowing it, into a more wholesome mental
atmosphere than that which she has been accustomed to breathe. The effect upon her general
health when this state of things can be obtained
will be marvelous. The nurse will need to remember that each patient offers her a new problem, and
that she must not attempt the same methods with
all.

CHAPTER XVI.

PREPARATIONS FOR GYNÆCOLOGICAL EXAMINATIONS.

The nurse is frequently called upon to aid the

History of disease. physician in obtaining a satisfactory history of a patient suspected of having pelvic trouble. The following plan is that generally adopted with us :—

1. A short sketch of the family history, health of parents, brothers and sisters ; if any deaths among them, their cause. These facts are of importance as showing a predisposition to any especial class of diseases.

2. The personal history of the patient, her health in childhood, the diseases from which she may then have suffered. Date of first menstruation, character as to existence of pain at periods ; amount of flow, regularity, etc. Date of marriage, number of pregnancies, number of miscarriages, number of labors, character of labors, character of convalescence. General health during marriage or since puberty.

3. History of the special disease from which the

patient may be suffering ; its onset, duration, character of symptoms, supposed cause, etc.

4. Present state of health, general appearance, character of functions, appetite, digestion, quantity of urine passed in 24 hours ; the urinalysis. Examination of chest organs, abdominal organs and pelvic organs (determined by physician).

5. Special examination with reference to tumor or existing disease.

Physical Examination.—The physical examination of the pelvic organs is much better conducted upon a table covered with a blanket, rug, or comfortable, and provided with a small pillow, than it can possibly be upon a bed or sofa. In this way one avoids the sinking of the body into the soft bed, and affords other facilities for a thorough investigation of the diseased parts. A sheet or blanket for covering the patient gives the desired protection from exposure.

When it is necessary to employ a bed a sewing-board, or the leaf of a dining-table slipped under the upper sheet and covering, gives a hard surface upon which the patient may lie.

The patient's clothing should be loose around the waist, all the waistbands being unbuttoned or untied, corsets removed, and all heavy skirts. She should lie on her back in a first examination, unless directed otherwise by the physician. If the abdomen is to be examined first, the patient's feet may be placed on a chair or stand, as she lies on the table, the knees should be well drawn up so that the abdominal walls may be relaxed. A sheet should be spread over the lower limbs, the loosened skirts being either drawn down under it or thrown back over the chest, in order to expose the abdomen. The sheet may be drawn up over the abdomen, after the clothing has been adjusted for examination, until the physician is ready to proceed to its inspection. The table should have been previously adjusted in front of a window admitting a strong light. At the foot of the table should be placed a chair for the physician, and to its right a stand or chair with a basin of warm water containing some antiseptic solution (bichloride of mercury 1-4000), soap and a towel.

Adjustment of patient. When the pelvic examination is to be made the limbs must be drawn up and separated, the feet resting on a level with the patient's buttocks. The patient's skirts are pushed up beneath the sheet until they rest over the abdomen, the sheet covers completely the lower limbs, pelvis, and abdomen.

Special tables and chairs. A variety of gynæcological tables and chairs exist. The nurse will have to be taught the management of any especial kind by the physician in whose office or hospital she may be called upon to work. In a private house an ordinary kitchen table

serves the purpose very well.   The chief advantage
of the special tables consists in the foot-rests, which
are so adjusted as to let the patient's hips be brought

FIG.˙ 51.

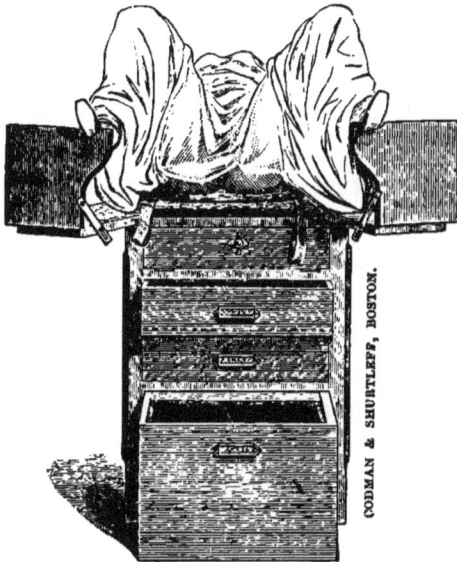

Chadwick's Gynæcological Table with Patient Arranged for
Examination.

well to the edge of the table, thus facilitating the
use of the speculum.

Should the patient be extremely nervous, or the
investigation involve much pain, it may be neces- Use of anæsthetic.
sary for an anæsthetic to be given.   This can only

13

be done with safety if the patient's stomach be empty. Therefore, it is well for the patient not to have taken any food for some hours before the ex-

Preparation of bowels and bladder. amination. The lower bowel should have been thoroughly emptied by an enema prior to the examination, and the patient should be required to void her urine. The condition of both these organs has much to do with success in an examination. It may be necessary, should there be difficulty in the voiding of urine, to use the catheter for the patient prior to the examination. This should always be done immediately after etherization, when the patient requires to be anæsthetized, as the taking of ether, which usually causes considerable nervous excitement, is apt to lead to an excessive secretion. When an abdominal or pelvic tumor of any size exists, the soft rubber catheter, English or French, should be used. When the urethra is somewhat tortuous, the English catheter is preferable, because of its greater resistance. The silver or glass catheter might do injury to the tissues, because of its inability to adapt itself to the changes in direction of the canal.

Instruments for gynæcological examinations. The instruments to be used by the physician in the course of the examination must be prepared and handed to him by the nurse.

These will be different forms of specula, as the bi-valve, the cylindrical and single blade speculum, the uterine dressing forceps, applicators, and, possibly, the uterine sound.

There are many varieties of specula named for Specula.

FIG. 52.

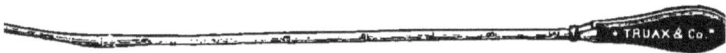

The Uterine Sound.

their respective inventors. Those most used are probably Cusco's bi-valve speculum, so called

FIG. 53.

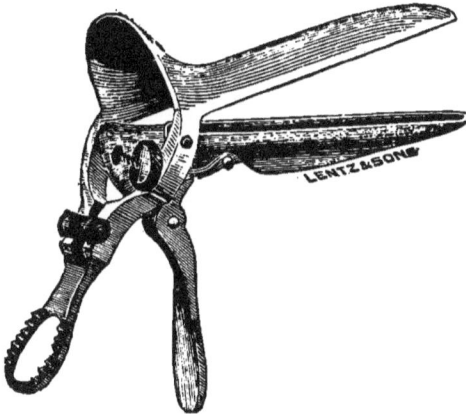

Bi-valve Speculum.

because of its having two blades. Fergusson's cylindrical speculum, made of clear glass, or glass silvered and covered with black varnish, so that it will act as a reflector.

FIG. 54.

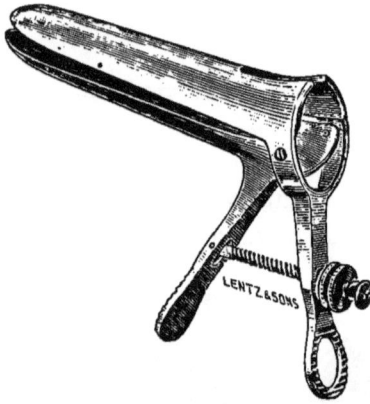

Small Bi-valve Speculum.

The cylindrical speculum may also be made of celluloid or hard rubber.

FIG. 55.

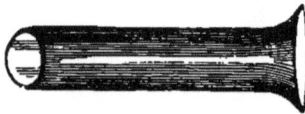

Fergusson's Speculum, Cylindrical.

The single blade speculum, sometimes called the duck-bill speculum, or Sims' speculum, has also many modifications.

It is not necessary to remember these by the names of their inventors, but rather to know them by their special characteristics.

Metallic specula are nickel-plated, as a rule. Material of which made. Recently aluminium, which is a very light metal, has been used in making them. Aluminium specula have, further, the advantage of not tarnishing or corroding when they come in contact with the

FIG. 56.

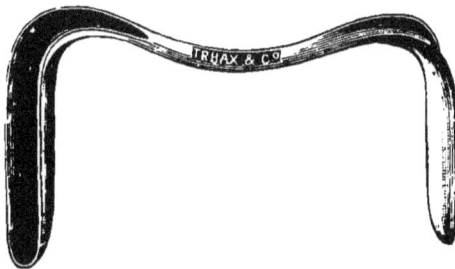

Sims' Speculum (Duck-bill).

chemical substances ordinarily used in making uterine applications. Bichloride of mercury will, however, corrode it, hence solutions of bichloride will need to be avoided in using this as other metallic instruments.

Nickel-plated instruments should not be rubbed Methods of cleaning. too vigorously or too frequently with sandsoap, whiting, etc., as the nickel wears off. The boiling or steaming of such instruments is the better way of cleansing them after use.

Dressing forceps.

The dressing forceps and sound are usually of metal (steel, nickel-plated), although the flexible

Applicators. sound may consist of rubber. Applicators, that is small rods for the carrying of cotton charged with some medicament to the neck or body of the uterus, may be of metal, rubber, or wood. A very convenient and inexpensive applicator for hospital use is the wooden splint about six inches long, which

FIG. 57.

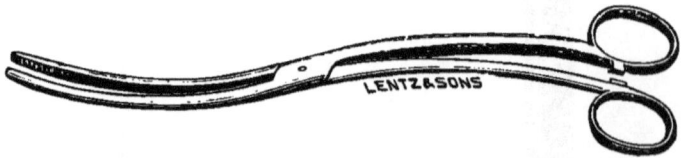

Dressing Forceps.

represents one stage in the process of the preparation of matches. These may be obtained in large quantities at match factories and kept with a little cotton twisted on one end for use as desired.

Preparation of instruments.

The instruments as required for use by the examining physician should be taken from a warm carbolized solution in which they have previously been placed; lubricated, if specula, with a little carbolized cosmoline, in order that they may slip without resistance into the vagina, rectum or urethra, and handed thus to the physician. After the speculum has been placed the nurse will need to hand the dressing forceps, between the extremities of which a little dry absorbent cotton may be held. This will be needed to cleanse the passage of any discharge which may obscure the view.

Similar pieces of cotton should be kept in readiness by the nurse, being placed as small twists or balls in a glass or china vessel within reach of the examiner, should more than the one be required.

A waste bucket or bowl should be placed beneath the foot of the table to receive waste matter.

Should the physician desire to make an application to the parts brought to view, the nurse may moisten the cotton on an applicator in a small quantity of the medicament specified by him, which should be poured out into a small china or glass vessel kept for the purpose. The cotton should not be saturated with the substance, as it may then drip over the tissues where not desired and produce unpleasant effects.

Should a tampon need to be placed, this should similarly be prepared by the nurse, caught between the blades of the dressing-forceps and handed to the physician.

Upon the removal of the speculum, and after having assisted the patient to alight from the table and dress, the nurse should give her attention to a thorough cleansing of the instruments used, particularly if they are to be immediately employed for another case.

They should be placed in warm water and scrubbed with nailbrush and soap. Should there be a steam sterilizer in operation in the room, they may then be dropped into it, until needed for the next patient. Ten minutes will suffice for their sterilization when the steam is at its height. In lieu of this, boiling water may be poured over them, or they may be placed in a 5 per cent carbolic solution until again needed. On taking instruments from so strong a carbolic solution, they should be rinsed in clear warm water before they are lubricated and handed to the physician for use, as they will otherwise cause the patient pain from the cauterant effect of the carbolic acid. Some physicians sterilize their instruments for office use by holding them in the flame of an alcohol lamp for a few minutes. Another duty of the nurse, in attend-

ance upon a physician making examinations, will be to place the patient in the positions desired. These positions are known as follows :—

The *lithotomy position,* is the ordinary recumbent position, the limbs being markedly flexed upon the abdomen. This is more commonly called for in certain operative procedures than during examination.   The method of maintaining it by the legstraps will be described later.

The *Sims position*, for bringing the uterine cervix within easy access, and for making rectal examinations.   The patient lies on her left side, with her left arm drawn behind her, so as to let her rest on

FIG. 58.

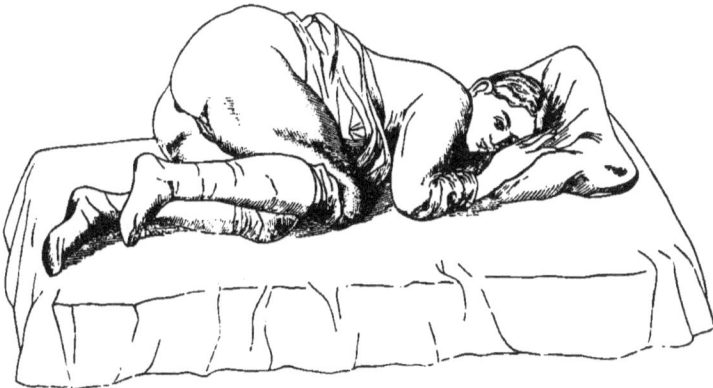

Sims' Position.

the left side of her chest.   The right leg should be so flexed as to let the right knee lie just above the left.   This position is necessary for the use of Sims' speculum.   The patient's clothing being well drawn up under her hips and a sheet thrown over the lower extremities for their protection, the physician introduces Sims' speculum, which the nurse holds in place with one hand, while with the other she lifts the right buttock to aid in the exposure of the vulvar orifice and vagina.

Genu-pectoral position.

The *knee-chest* position is one which is frequently assumed for the replacement of the pelvic organs, or the appreciation of their mobility.

FIG. 59.

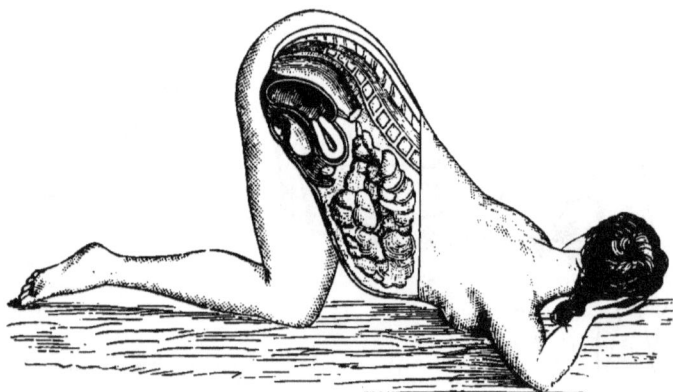

Genu-pectoral Position.

This is obtained by having the patient place herself upon her knees, and bend forward so that her chest may rest on a pillow placed upon the bed or table, her head resting beyond the pillow on one side or the other. The arms should be placed in an extended position at her side or may be clasped around the sides of the table, so that she may not be tempted to rest upon her elbows. This brings the hips to a point considerably above the head, and enables the abdominal and pelvic organs to gravitate towards the diaphragm. The patient's clothing should be pushed back from under her knees and lifted above her hips, the sheet being draped over her for the protection of the parts thus uncovered. A separation of the buttocks by the hands will allow of the entrance of air into the vagina, which will serve to force the pelvic organs forward.

In cases of displacement of the uterus the nurse may be called upon to assist the patient to take this position several times daily.

CHAPTER XVII.

PREPARATIONS FOR GYNÆCOLOGICAL OPERATIONS

The divisions of this subject may be classified as follows :—

1. Preparation of the room.
2. Preparation of the sponges, instruments, etc.
3. Preparation of the patient.
4. Preparation of operator and assistants.
5. Nurse's duty during operation and convalescence.

PREPARATION OF THE ROOM.

Excepting for vaginal hysterectomy (removal of the uterus through the vagina), which is to be regarded as a major operation, it will not be necessary to remove carpets, furniture, etc., from a room which is clean and thoroughly well kept. It is well, however, in any operation to have special provision made for the protection of the floor.

Protection for floor.

Prior to the operation the room should be thoroughly swept and dusted, and well aired. Superfluous furniture and hangings, because they interfere with ventilation, it is always desirable to

remove. All operations are better done on a table
than on the bed. Therefore one should be prepared by the nurse. As in operations on the pelvic
organs the patient will have to lie with her hips
close to the edge of the table, the knees being
drawn up, one table, of the ordinary size of a
kitchen table, will be sufficient, without the table
placed transversely to this for the head, as in abdominal section.

The table should be placed before a window, so
that there may be thoroughly good light. Some
protective, as a piece of oil-cloth or drugget, should
be spread under it. The arrangement of the dressings for the table should be the same as described
for abdominal section—a blanket or comfortable
spread over the table and tacked down round the
edges. A piece of rubber should protect this
covering, at least over the lower half of the table,
when the operating pad is not used. A sheet
should be spread over these and similarly fastened
down at the sides. A blanket and sheet for covering the patient, and a pillow protected with rubber
cloth fastened around it, under the slip, should be
arranged on the table. A chair should be placed
at the foot of the table for the operator. The
stand for his instruments should be placed to his
right, within easy reach. On this stand should
also be found a tray or vessel containing a steril-

ized solution for him to dip his instruments into while in use, or to use in cleansing his hands, from time to time, of blood.

Two assistants usually stand one on each side of the table, to aid the operator by holding the patient's limbs in any desired position, also in aiding with instruments, ligatures, sponging, etc. The nurse with her table for cleansing the sponges should stand back of the assistant on the operator's left, handing him sponges and receiving them from him for recleansing. Her stand should contain one basin filled with cold sterilized water for washing out the blood, and another basin with warm sterilized water for keeping them in until needed.

A chair or stool should be placed at the side of the table to aid the patient in stepping up. The window should be screened from the outside gaze by a thin lace or muslin curtain, or a sheet of newspaper may be pinned across it. A waste bucket should stand under the table immediately in front of the operator. The operating pad may be placed at the lower edge of the table so that its flap rests over the waste bucket and thus conducts the water used in irrigation, etc., into it.

When the operator works without a pad it is well to have a folded sheet so placed over the lower portion of the table as to extend from beneath the patient's hips over the lap of the operator.

This serves to protect the operator's clothing, the
floor at the foot of the table, etc., from soiling.

The bed for the reception of the patient after The bed.

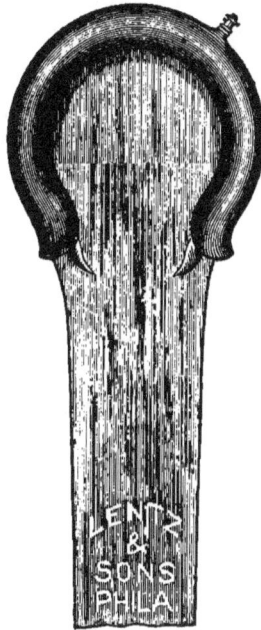

FIG. 60.

Operating Pad.

operation should be arranged beforehand.   It
should be so placed that access may be had to it
on three sides.   It should not face the light.   A
firm mattress, as of hair, is the most desirable.

Care should be taken to see that the bed is in every way comfortable. A pad should protect the mattress, and a rubber protective should be so placed over this as to cover the portion of the bed, over which the parts operated upon shall rest. In pelvic operations this will be the middle of the bed, in a breast operation the upper part of the bed. A sheet is spread over these, and a draw-sheet, that is, a sheet folded upon itself twice in its length, is fastened over the portion of the bed beneath which the protective has been placed.

Warming
the bed. A heated soapstone or hot-water bag should be placed, previous to the operation, between the upper and lower bedclothes, so that the bed may be warm for the reception of the patient.

Antiseptic
solutions. The nurse should learn before the operation the kind of solutions to be used, if antiseptic solutions are to be employed. Should bichloride of mercury and carbolic acid be employed, which are the usual solutions desired by surgeons, a large bottle containing a solution of 1–500 or 1–1000 of the former and another containing 1–20 of the latter will enable the weaker solutions to be prepared with great rapidity. Thus, if a solution of 1–4000 of the bichloride be called for, the nurse taking one part of the 1–1000 (as one gill) can add three parts (or three gills) of warm sterilized water to this, thus obtaining a warm solution of the required proportion. If a bath thermometer be kept in the Regulating the tempe- rature of solutions. basin during the admixture of the solution and the water, the nurse may, by watching the column of mercury, determine whether to make the addition from the warm or cold water, until she obtains the quantity desired.

A solution of 1–1000 can be prepared by mixing Methods for quick preparation of solutions. in equal parts the solution 1–500 and warm sterilized water.

A solution of 1–40 carbolic acid (that usually employed for the immersion of instruments) may be made by adding the same quantity of warm sterilized water to a solution of 1–20.

Sometimes surgeons prefer the use of tablets of bichloride in making up solutions. The directions as to the strength of one of these will be found upon the vial in each case. As a rule, a tablet represents 7½ grs., which, when added to a pint of water, gives a solution of 1–1000. A fountain syringe containing the solution to be used should be filled and hung behind and considerably above the operator, on a nail, that it may be ready when needed.

When the operator is obliged to use the edge Arrange- ments when operation done on bed. of a bed in place of a table, the bed should be placed with one side sufficiently near the window to obtain a good light. The sinking of the patient in the bed may be prevented by placing a board

14

beneath the mattress and the springs, or between the mattress and pad. This portion of the bed should then be arranged for the operation in the same way that the table was arranged as to the protective rubber and sheet.

A chair or stool of proper height with reference to the bed should be placed in front of this arrangement. The floor, for about one foot beneath the bed, on that side, and extending to at least two feet beyond it, should be protected by floor oilcloth or old carpeting.

Prepara-
tion of
sponges,
etc.

The stands and other articles required should be arranged as before described. The preparation of sponges and instruments for the operation will be identical with those described in the chapter on the subject of their preparation for abdominal section. The dressings employed will vary somewhat as to their character, form, etc., with the choice of the operator.

T-bandage
and anti-
septic pad.

For operations upon the floor of the pelvis, or within the vagina, a T-bandage with an antiseptic pad of some kind will be necessary. The T-bandage will consist of a straight abdominal bandage of firm muslin, to which a strip of muslin about four inches wide is fastened at right angles, so that it may serve as a perineal band passing between the limbs and fastened before and behind to the lower edge of the abdominal bandage.

A folded towel or napkin, pinned by a safety-pin to the abdominal bandage, serves the purpose very well.

The antiseptic pad is usually made of one of the different kinds of antiseptic gauze, in which anti-septic jute, oakum, or cotton may be enclosed.

In the Woman's Hospital the Garrigues' "Oc- Occlusion dressing. clusion Dressing," somewhat modified, similar to that used for obstetric work in the Maternity connected with the Hospital, has been employed.

This consists of one or more pieces of dry patent lint, 6 x 8 inches, which have previously been rendered antiseptic by saturation in a solution of bichloride of mercury 1–1000.

These are placed over the vulva, doubled in their width so as to make a dressing 3 x 8 inches. The lint is then covered by a piece of gutta-percha tissue, 4 x 9 inches, which is wet in a 1–4000 solution of bichloride of mercury.

These dressings are kept in place by a napkin of sublimated cheese-cloth, 18 inches square, folded to form a diagonal 5 inches in width, within whose folds a pad of oakum is enclosed. The napkin is tightly fastened to an abdominal bandage, both anteriorly and posteriorly by means of safety pins and the access of air to the vagina is thus prevented. These dressings are changed as they may require, according to the amount of discharge. Should the catheter have to be used at stated intervals, fresh dressings should be employed in again protecting the parts.

The nurse can obtain the cheese-cloth at any drygoods store, and prepare it by first thoroughly washing with softsoap and boiling, and then wringing it out in a solution of bichloride of mercury 1–1000. The patent lint, obtained in a drug store, may be rendered antiseptic in the same way. The gutta-percha tissue and oakum may also be obtained at a drug store, the former more advantageously, perhaps, at a rubber store, where also a good syringe should be obtained for use in the case, if required.

Although bichloride gauze is most commonly used, iodoform gauze may be preferred by some surgeons.

The preparation of ligatures and sutures, the threading of needles, etc., does not usually devolve upon the nurse, yet may be required of her. The same rules must be observed as in their preparation for abdominal operations. The needles vary much in size and shape, according to the character of the operation to be done. The surgeon, too, will have his own choice as to the kind of needle he prefers. The nurse must, therefore, learn his preference and observe it.

A sterilized towel, containing a set of dressings

neatly folded, the bandage, safety-pins and box of iodoform powder to be used in the dressing of the wound, should be brought to the surgeon by the nurse at the proper time for their application, hence should be kept in readiness.

CHAPTER XVIII.

PREPARATION OF THE PATIENT, OPERATOR, AND ASSISTANTS.

A good mental condition.

First of all it is important to get the patient into a good mental condition. She should have her thoughts, so far as possible, kept off the operation. The utmost tact will be necessary to manage this successfully.

It is well to make all the preparations for operation elsewhere than in the presence of the patient.

Preparation of bowels.

If the operation is to be on the pelvic organs, involving vagina, uterus, bladder, or rectum, it will be especially necessary to have a thorough evacuation of the bowels. The night before the operation a laxative or purgative may be given, and the morning following; the lower bowel may be further cleansed by an injection of soap and water.

Abstinence from food.

The patient should not have any breakfast on the morning of the operation. If the operation is not to be done before noon, she may receive a cup of coffee or tea, or a cup of beef-tea early in the morning.

Rest.

She should remain in bed, lest she should feel faint for want of food.

A full bath should have been taken on the night Bath. previous to operation. She should wear, according to the weather, a merino or gauze vest, a pair of Clothing. drawers and stockings, a long nightdress. When the vest is worn a chemise should be dispensed with, as it is an awkward garment to remove when a change is needed, especially where the patient must be kept as quiet as possible. The hair should Arrangement of be parted in the back and plaited in two braids, one hair. behind each ear. This is most convenient when lying upon the back, and prevents matting of hair.

A vaginal injection of bichloride of mercury or Vaginal injection. some other disinfectant will probably need to be given just before the operation. The vulva and Cleansing and disinfection of surrounding parts will need especial preparation by vulva. a thorough cleansing, first with soap and warm water and then with some disinfectant solutions. The hair about the vulva is often shaved up to a Shaving of parts. level with the "meatûs urinarius," or entrance to the bladder. The choice of the surgeon regarding the shaving should be learned by the nurse previous to her attempting the same. Many surgeons prefer attending to the especial preparation of the site of operation after etherization.

In private houses the anæsthetic is generally Administration of administered in an adjoining room, and the patient the anæsthetic. afterward carried in and placed upon the operating table. The nurse aids the surgeon in carrying out these arrangements. She should learn from him in what position the patient is desired when placed upon the table. The dorsal position—the patient lying upon her back with the limbs flexed— is that usually required for operations upon the vagina or the perineum. The patient's clothing in

FIG. 61.

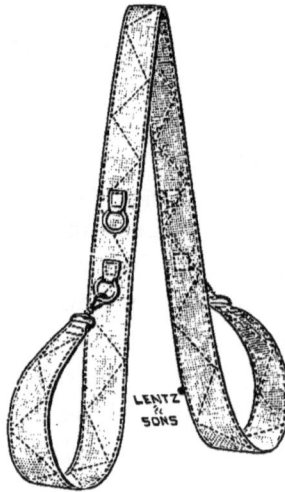

Leg-holder.

this position should be well drawn up from under the hips and pushed above the operating pad, which is then placed under her. The limbs being flexed may be fixed in position by the leg-holder, as shown in the cut, or held by assistants. The leg-holder being thrown around the patient's neck is fastened, just above the knee, to each limb.

A sheet should be so draped over the person as to cover the limbs and protect the patient so far as possible from unnecessary exposure.

A double fold of sterilized gauze, about a yard square, with a slit cut in it, through which the

FIG. 62.

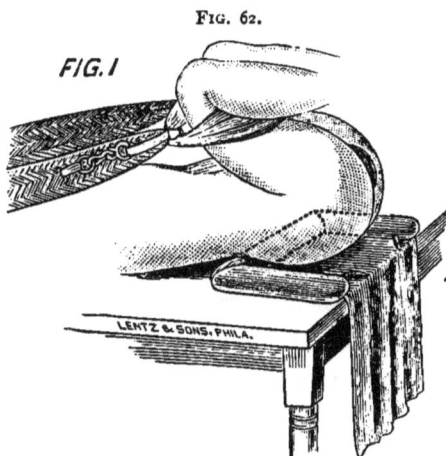

Dorsal Position and Arrangement for Operations on Floor of Pelvis.

special site of operation may be exposed, is used by some surgeons as a further protection against exposure, being draped from beneath the sheet over the vulva and buttocks, the operator carrying on his manipulations through the opening which exposes the special site to be operated upon.

Sims' position.

The Sims position is frequently used in cervical operations, for fistulæ, or for operations about the anus, as for hemorrhoids.

"Genu-pectoral" position.

The knee-chest position is but seldom used for operation except in certain forms of fistulæ. The patient's chest in such cases may need to be supported by a thick pillow or a padded stool, to bring her into proper position for the operator.

The nurse should in every case aim to keep the patient's clothing out of the way of the operator, and from contact with the discharges, but she should so adjust sheets, towels, etc., as to save the patient any unnecessary exposure.

Preparation of operator and assistants.

The preparation of the operator and assistants will be practically the same as that observed in preparation for abdominal section.

Any open surface upon the patient's body may become a source of infection, therefore the requirements of asepsis and antisepsis should be as rigidly observed as possible in the preparations for any operative procedure.

CHAPTER XIX.

DUTIES OF NURSE DURING OPERATION.

The patient being placed, and the operation begun, the nurse, unless directed otherwise, will need Attention to sponges. to station herself by the stand which contains the vessels for cleansing the sponges. Several "mounted "Mounted sponges." sponges" should be prepared, that is, sponges cut about the size of a walnut, placed on stems of metal or rubber, called sponge-holders. Forceps with catches may be used when these are not on hand.

For operations in the vagina or on the cervix, etc., these mounted sponges are especially necessary.

The nurse, while attending to the sponges, especially, should be ready to respond to any demand Attention to surgeon's needs. of the surgeon—changing the water in the basins, Changing of solutions in basins. refilling the irrigator, removing soiled towels and Cleansing of her own hands. replacing them with fresh. Her own hands should be carefully cleansed after each of these services, in a basin containing some antiseptic solution, as 1–4000 bichloride of mercury, before she again touches the sponges.

The sponges should be thoroughly cleansed of

Management of sponges. blood in the basin of cold water and allowed to lie in warm water until wanted. They should be squeezed until as free of moisture as possible, and should be handed in quick succession to the assistant nearest to her who will have the sponging to attend to.

Avoidance of curiosity. At no time in any operation should the nurse allow herself to become so engrossed in watching the operation as to forget that there are duties Attention to duty. incumbent upon her. She should give her sole attention to the performance of her own duties, and no more think of watching the operation (except as she may need to do so for the proper appreciation of the special duties that may devolve upon her at each step), than should the etherizer, whose sole attention should be engrossed in the proper performance of his work.

Duties at completion of operation. At the completion of the operation, the nurse may assist in slipping the rubber pad from beneath the patient. It may be placed in the waste bucket temporarily, while she proceeds with a sponge and a dry sterilized towel to prepare the parts for the Application of dressings. application of the dressings. When entirely dry the powder, boric acid, or iodoform may be applied by the surgeon, and then the dressings are put in place and fastened down by a bandage. A blanket Removal of patient to bed. is then wrapped around the patient and she may be lifted into the bed which the nurse, just before the application of the dressings, should have prepared for her reception, by turning down the covers and removing temporarily the hot soapstone or water-bag.   The latter may then be replaced at the patient's feet; a soft towel should have been placed, in lieu of a pillow, under the patient's head and another towel should be placed under her chin.   A light basin for the patient to vomit in, in case she is sick, should be placed under the head of the bed; a chair for the doctor should be placed beside the bed.   While the doctor and his assistant give their attention to the patient, the nurse may quickly remove all the articles used during the operation.

Application of warmth.

Further attentions.

Removal of articles used during operations.

CHAPTER XX.

SPECIAL NURSING IN GYNÆCOLOGICAL OPERATIONS.

Points of difference in management of cases.

There will be little points of difference in the management of each case, which will depend upon the character of the operation performed. Some of the most frequent gynæcological operations will therefore be referred to separately, in order that the especial points in their nursing may be demonstrated.

Immediate attentions after operation.

After minor operations there is seldom the profound shock which exists after an abdominal or any other major operation. Should there be, the nurse will need to give her attention to the restoration of the patient, as has already been described in the treatment after abdominal section.

Cleaning of room.

Should the nurse not be needed by the patient, the doctor or his assistants remaining for a short time with her, the nurse may quietly and quickly busy herself with removing the operating table, soiled sheets, towels, etc., and setting the room in order. When the doctor leaves, her place is by her patient.

Exact directions.

Careful directions should be received by her as

222

to her especial duties in each case. She should inquire of the surgeon whether the patient may be permitted to have her position changed from time to time; what shall be done concerning the use of the catheter; the amount of nourishment given the patient; the use of any medicines, etc. These facts should be carefully put down on paper and kept for her guidance in the care of the case.

Rupture of the perineum is so frequent that the operation for its repair, known as the "perineal operation," is the most common of the gynæcological operations. The extent of the laceration which is usually the result of childbirth varies. When it extends through the sphincter muscle of the bowel it is called a complete rupture.

It is not only important in the repair of these injuries that the operation should be well done, but that the healing of the wound should in every way be promoted. The patient's general health should, therefore, be in a satisfactory condition, and the bowels should have received very careful attention for several days. When we remember that the intestinal canal is about twenty-five feet long, and that fæcal masses are often kept stored up in it for months, we can understand how free evacuations on several successive days may be necessary before the patient is in fit condition for operation. Some laxative, as recommended by the physician in

Perineorrhaphy for rupture of perineum.

Complete rupture.

Preparatory treatment for operation.

The bowels.

charge of the case, will be necessary during this period. The opening of the bowels twice every twenty-four hours is not too frequent. An enema will need to be administered a few hours before operation. Care should be taken not to set up a diarrhœa, as this condition may cause greater inconvenience than constipation during the convalescence. The preparatory treatment will also

Hemor-
rhoids.

include attention to hemorrhoids, if they exist, or discharges from the uterus and vagina. When hemorrhoids exist, it is well to keep them supported by a T-bandage, and a compress over the anus.

Vaginal
discharges.

Discharges from the vagina, which may interfere with healing, must be cured before the operation is undertaken. The use of hot-water injections, given by the nurse, and local treatment as required by the physician, will be necessary for this.

Position
during
operation.

For the operation the patient will need to be placed in the lithotomy or dorsal position. The preparations for fixing her in this position should, of course, not be undertaken until she is fully etherized and no longer in a condition to be frightened by them.

Special ar-
rangements
for opera-
tion.

Her limbs may then be flexed upon the abdomen and held either by an assistant on each side, or by the legholder. The clothing under her back being well pushed up, the hips are brought to the edge of the table and the operating pad adjusted beneath them.   The parts are washed thoroughly, first with soap and water and then an antiseptic solution, and the hair on the posterior part of the vulva and the perineum shaved away or cut close. Sterilized sheets or towels are made to envelope the limbs and protect the parts.   A large pan or foot-tub should lie just below the parts on the floor, so as to catch blood or water used in irrigation.   The labia are held apart by the assistants on each side.   The fingers of one hand of each of the assistants can hold back these greater lips, while the other hand of each remains free to assist with sponges, holding instruments, etc.   The assistants should stand so as to keep out of the operator's light.   The nurse attends to cleansing and handing the sponges, changing the water in the basins, and responding to the needs of surgeon and assistants.   After the completion of the operation a T-bandage with antiseptic dressings, as before *Application of dressings.* described, may be applied or not, according to the wish of the surgeon, and the patient placed in bed. The knees and thighs are flexed, and she is put *After-care.* to bed on the right or left side, as a rule, although many surgeons now put little stress upon position as important in the after-management of their cases. Some surgeons prefer that the patient should continue to lie on her side, her position being made

15

comfortable by pillows, until a day or two after removal of sutures.

The external parts will, from time to time, require washing, as a rule, as there is sometimes a little discharge. The washing may be accomplished by means of a stream of tepid antiseptic solution, as bichloride of mercury 1–4000, or 1–40 of carbolic acid, from a syringe, and the parts then carefully dried with a piece of antiseptic lint or gauze. If there is no discharge, the parts should simply be kept dry. A powder, as boric acid or iodoform, may be dusted over the site of the wound from time to time, to insure this. The vagina will only need to be washed out, should there be a discharge. Great care must be taken in the insertion of the nozzle that no injury is done to the stitches. It should be seen that the water returns freely from the vagina. Pressing the nozzle of the syringe against the anterior wall of the vagina will be apt to leave space enough for the return current.

Catheterization. The catheter may need to be used every six or eight hours for several days. A loaded bladder makes the patient restless. Some surgeons prefer having the patient pass her water from the first. There is probably little, if any, danger of urine irritating the wound. Should the urine be passed, the parts should be afterward irrigated with an antiseptic solution and thoroughly and carefully dried.

The use of the catheter, unless aseptically carried out, may cause irritation of the bladder, which is often a source of great suffering.

The question of opening the bowels is very important, especially in cases of complete rupture. The practice of surgeons differs in this respect. Some keep the bowels locked for a week or ten days, by the administration of opiates. The usual practice, however, is to keep the bowels free from the first, as the hard masses (scybala) which are apt to form put the united parts to great danger, from the strain to which they subject them. *Time and method for securing an action of the bowels.*

If the bowels have not been moved by the fourth day, the practice is to administer a gill of cotton-seed oil by bowel, allowing it to remain while laxatives are administered by mouth, as a teaspoonful of castor-oil every hour, until four to six doses have been taken, or the bowels feel like moving. The dose of oil may be administered in a half a Seidlitz powder, flavored with a drop of oil of peppermint, or gaultheria, or a little syrup of ginger, etc. This prevents the nausea attendant usually upon taking the oil. By this method, a soft evacuation of the bowels is secured, and, if the precaution be taken to have the patient lie on her side while the bowels are moved, there will be little injurious effect from strain. A thorough irrigation and cleansing and drying of the parts should follow. Should *Subsequent cleansing.*

Relief from flatus.

the patient be disturbed by flatus before the bowels are moved, having a bearing down sensation with pain, an English catheter, about No. 9 or 10, may be insinuated into the bowel and thus aid the escape of gas.

Diet

The diet of the patient for 24 to 48 hours should be simply milk, broth, or beef-tea, and this with farinaceous foods should be given until about the fifth or sixth day, when meat should be given.

The deep perineal sutures, or stitches, should be removed in about eight or ten days. The rectal sutures do not always require removal. The nurse will need to place the patient across the bed for the purpose, drawing her hips close to its edge, and flexing the limbs. Her limbs should be protected by slipping on a pair of drawers and stockings. A sheet should in addition be thrown over her and draped around the limbs. A sheet or napkin should be placed under her hips.

A chair for the surgeon should be placed in front of the patient, and a sheet or towel thrown over his knees as he takes his seat.

As the surgeon usually desires to give a vaginal injection before removing the stitches, if he has not directed the nurse to attend to giving this injection herself, she should have in readiness the antiseptic solution required, a syringe, and a bedpan. The instruments, straight, sharp-pointed scissors and a

pair of anatomical forceps, should be placed in a
tin basin and immersed in a carbolic solution 1–40.
An antiseptic solution, as 1–4000 of bichloride of
mercury, should be prepared in a china or agate
basin for the doctor's hands.

A pus-pan or piece of paper for receiving the
stitches as removed should be placed on the bed,
within convenient reach of the surgeon.   The nurse

FIG. 63.

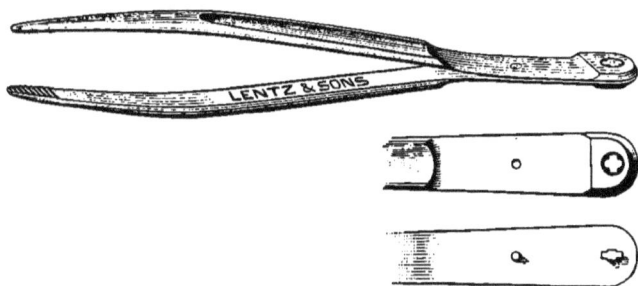

Aseptic Anatomical Forceps.
The two branches being separable are more readily cleansed.

should then support the patient's limbs, or, if there
are other assistants to do this, she will assist the surgeon in giving the douche, and in obtaining for him
or handing him the various articles required as he
needs them.   After the removal of the stitches she
assists in putting the patient properly back in bed
and removes the articles which were used in the
operation.

Removal of sutures.

Necessity for quiet after sutures removed. The patient will need to be kept quiet, as a rule, for a day or two after the removal of the stitches. The nurse should, however, always learn from the surgeon his special wishes concerning the subsequent management of a case.

Operation for partial rupture of perineum. In partial rupture of the perineum the management is practically the sameas in complete rupture, except that there will be less fear of damage when the bowels are opened on the third or fourth day, and that the stitches are usually removed at the end of a week.

The operation for repair of the perineum is known as perineorraphy. The various methods of doing this operation are known by the names of their different inventors.

Elytror-rhaphy or Polpor-rhaphy. Elytrorrhaphy or colporrhaphy are commonly known as "vaginal operations," that is, operations on the vagina for the relief of prolapsus, or falling of the womb.

After-treatment. The after-treatment is much the same as in cases where rupture of the perineum has been repaired. The patient will need to lie in bed for over two weeks, and the bladder must never be allowed to become distended, or the cicatrix will be stretched Removal of sutures. or broken down. The sutures are removed from the tenth to the fifteenth day. The patient will need to avoid active exercise for many months.

Trachelorrhaphy is an operation done for the repair of the cervix or neck of the womb, when Trachelor-rhaphy or cervical operation. laceration exists. It is frequently spoken of as a "cervical operation." Before this operation is performed, the surgeon generally has the patient put upon preparatory treatment for a week or two, to Preparatory treatment. remove all tenderness and congestion. Hot water injections daily, sometimes several times a day, are ordered, after which the doctor may apply tampons of glycerine, etc.

Some surgeon's prefer the semi-prone or Sims' The operation. position for this operation, as this enables the neck of the womb to be brought within easy reach. The operation is more frequently performed with the patient on her back, in what is called the dorsal or lithotomy position.

The patient should remain in bed a fortnight or Rest in bed. more after the operation and remain in the recumbent position so that there may be no strain upon the stitches. Some counter-irritant, as burning fluid, is frequently applied on cotton over the lower part of the abdomen. The bowels should not be The bowels. allowed to get constipated, a movement being secured by means of laxatives daily or every other day.

The patient's diet need not be restricted. After Diet. the second day, especially if there be much discharge, a vaginal injection of tepid water, contain- Vaginal injections. ing some antiseptic (as bichloride of mercury

1–4000), may be employed. After urine has been passed or the catheter used, it is also well to use a warm-water injection to avoid irritation of the wound through urine which may pass into the vagina.

Removal of sutures. The sutures are sometimes removed as early as the seventh day. The patient is placed in Sims' position for this, and the nurse will have to hold the speculum and support the right buttock, the patient lying on her left side, and *vice versâ* when she lies on her right side, while the surgeon removes the stitches. More frequently the sutures are not removed until the fourteenth day, or even **After-care.** later. The patient should be kept quiet for some days after the removal of the stitches, not even sitting up in bed. This is to give time for the cicatrix to grow stronger. The nurse will, of course, observe the wishes of the surgeon in this as in other matters pertaining to the nursing.

Operations for fistulæ. Operations for fistulæ are not infrequent. A fistula is an unnatural opening produced by sloughing of the tissues. It may be the result of cancer, but in operable cases is more frequently the result of child-birth. The constant pressure of a pessary worn too long may cause it. An opening may in this way be formed between the bladder and the **Varieties of fistulæ.** vagina, in which case it is called a vesico-vaginal fistula, or it may be formed between the bowel and the vagina, when it is called a recto-vaginal fistula.

Constant dribbling of the urine is occasioned by *Symptoms.* the former condition, while escape of fæces through the vagina is a result of the latter.

The lithotomy position is that usually employed *Method of conducting examination.* in doing the operation, or examining for the condition. A Sims speculum retracts the perineum. When it is difficult to detect the fistula, warm milk may be injected into the bladder or rectum, and the vagina watched to discover where it makes its exit. This will betray the position of the fistula.

Should a fistula occur as the result of a difficult *Spontaneous healing.* delivery, it is possible that, if at once discovered and properly treated, it may heal without an operation. The vagina should be kept perfectly clean *Precautions to be observed.* by frequent syringing with warm antiseptic solutions, and a self-retaining catheter should be placed in the bladder and the latter thus kept empty.

In performing the operation for vesico-vaginal *Operation for vesico-vaginal fistula.* fistula the surgeon will have the patient placed in the position he may prefer—the lithotomy, the semi-prone, or the genu-pectoral. The lithotomy position is usually employed. The bowels should *Preparations.* be thoroughly cleared out by a laxative administered about forty-eight hours before the operation, and an enema an hour or two before the operation

The patient's limb may be held by the leg-holder, the hips being placed over the operating pad. When all the stitches have been tied, the vagina and the bladder may be washed out with warm water (sterilized). If water is found to escape from the bladder into the vagina from the site of the wound, the operator will need to insert more After-care. stitches. After the operation a self-retaining catheter must be placed in the bladder to keep the urine drawn off. Some operators do not employ this. The catheter usually employed is the short

FIG. 64.

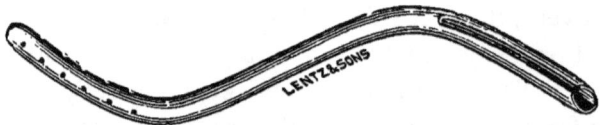

S-shaped Catheter.

catheter with a bulbous extremity to prevent its The self-retaining catheter. slipping out of the bladder. The sigmoid or S-shaped catheter requires more frequent removal for cleansing, and is more apt to do injury upon its withdrawal and introduction, which must be done daily for cleansing it. The upper curve of the S is intended to hold the catheter in place by resting against the pubic bone. The bulbous catheter may be made of hard rubber or vulcanite, and will need occasional removal for cleansing purposes.

It is best washed in a strong solution of acetic acid.

After the operation the patient is placed in bed, Position in bed. on her left side.   When a catheter has been introduced as described, a coach-urinal or a bedpan should be placed in the bed, behind the bent knees, which should be fastened together by means of a bandage.   A piece of flexible rubber tubing is Arrangement for drawing off urine. fitted on to the catheter at one end, the other being passed into the urinal.   When the patient is permitted to lie upon her back, the receptacle for

FIG. 65.

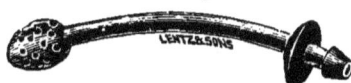

Bulbous Catheter.

the urine will need to be placed beneath her limbs. It is more liable to be pushed out of place in this position.   The nurse must frequently empty and cleanse the receptacle, to keep the bed free from odor.   The bowels must be kept in good condition, The bowels. no hard masses being allowed to collect in them, so as to cause irritation.   No straining effort should be permitted.   The fæcal masses, if they exist, may be softened by the injection of a gill of warm cotton-seed oil, in three or four hours a pint and a half of soap and water may be injected.   Should several hours elapse and the enema be retained, it is a good plan to introduce a tube (as the long vaginal nozzle) to the extent of about four inches, letting the outer end rest over a soap dish containing a little water. The tube, if left thus ten or twenty minutes, will usually carry off a quantity of flatus, and then the patient will, as a rule, have a free motion. Should the first enema prove unavailing, the process may be repeated.

Before the stitches are removed, a free evacuation of the bowels should be obtained, and the vagina

Removal of sutures.

cleansed with an antiseptic solution. The sutures are removed about the eighth or tenth day. The patient is placed in the semi-prone position and Sims' speculum used. For this process, the patient is best placed on a table, as a good light is required. Some of the complications which may occur after this operation are as follows:—

Hemorrhage into the bladder.

Hemorrhage into the bladder—perhaps the most common accident—is shown by the color of the urine drained off, and, if managed in the beginning by injections of warm water, can thus be usually checked. If irritation of the bladder, however, persists, and it is found that the bladder is distended, yet nothing can be drawn off by the catheter, the distention must be due to clots, and the

Secondary operation.

surgeon may have to reopen the fistula and remove the clots. Sometimes severe pain occurs extending

from the kidney on one side down to the blad- Closure of
ureter.
der. This symptom should be carefully reported,
as it may imply that a ureter has been closed, and
the removal of some stitches may be necessary.

Cystitis, or inflammation of the bladder, is often Cystitis.
a serious complication, as it leads to pain and a
constant desire to empty the bladder, hence straining efforts which may prevent the healing of the
fistula. The bladder may need to be washed out Management.
frequently with warm water, containing boric acid
or chlorate of potash, and the self-retaining catheter cannot be worn. The surgeon will attend to
the process of washing out the bladder, and the
nurse should not attempt it unless directed by him.
Warm poultices over the lower part of the abdomen, and flaxseed tea or other diluents may
need to be administered. Thus a tumblerful of
flaxseed tea may be administered once in three or
four hours.

In recto-vaginal fistula the operation is conducted Operation
for recto-
on the same principle as when a vesico-vaginal fis- vaginal
fistula.
tula is treated. The bowels must be thoroughly
cleaned out by an aperient administered twenty-
four hours before operation, followed by an enema
an hour or two before the patient is placed upon the
table.

A rectal tube or large-sized English catheter will
need to be retained in the bowel after operation, to

carry off flatus. The rules for after-treatment will be the same as in repair of complete rupture of the perineum. The chief trouble will consist in deciding as to the time when the bowels may be moved with safety. Efforts should be made to secure a soft movement, by means of the oil enema, as already described.

Removal of urethral caruncle. The removal of urethral caruncle is another operation very frequently performed. The caruncle is a small, sensitive tumor, sometimes of quite a bright red color, which is found at the entrance to the urethra. It causes pain and difficulty on urination, hence should be removed. When such growths cause no unpleasant symptoms, as is occasionally the case, it is not necessary to disturb them.

The operation. The patient for this operation should be placed in the lithotomy position, and the urine drawn off after she has been etherized.

Management of Paquelin's cautery. The Paquelin thermo-cautery is frequently used to sear the bleeding surface left by the removal of the tumor. The nurse may be called upon to prepare the cautery and have it in readiness. The finest point being fitted to the handle, it should be allowed to rest over the flame of an alcohol lamp until well heated. The rubber bulb at the end of the tube may then be compressed repeatedly and rather rapidly by the nurse until the point of the

cautery becomes red hot.   The vial containing
benzine should be kept at a safe distance from the
lamp and from the red-hot point, as the fluid is
inflammable.   The vial is usually provided with a

FIG. 66.

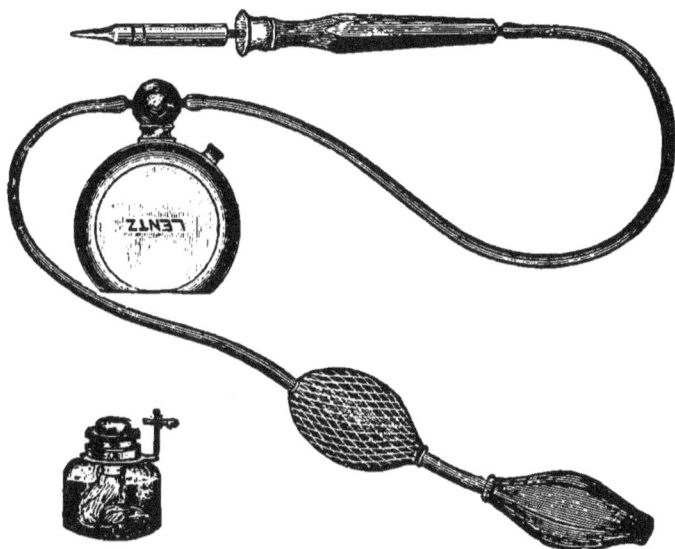

Thermo-Cautery (Paquelin's).

hook, by which it may be fastened to a button-hole
in the waist of the nurse's dress.   One hand is then
free for compression of the bulb and the other
holds the cautery by its wooden handle.   When
the point of the cautery is red hot it may be re-

moved from the flame of the lamp and the heat kept up by compression of the bulb, which forces the vapor of the benzine into contact with the lower portion of the cautery. When the point seems to be getting cold rapid compression of the bulb will again heat it up.

After the surgeon has finished with the use of the cautery it should be heated to a white heat by rapid compression of the bulb and the tubing pulled off the handle while it is still hot. This sudden cooling helps to preserve the point. The same instrument will sometimes be needed in the treatment of hemorrhoids—also for cauterizing the stump in abdominal section.

After-treatment.

The after-treatment in a case of urethral caruncle is very simple. The patient should be kept quiet in bed for a few days, and the urine should be drawn off about once in six hours for the first day, after which the patient may pass it. It may not be necessary to use the catheter at all, should the patient be able to pass her water from the first.

The use of some diluent drink will also aid in making the passage of urine less painful.

Operations for hemorrhoids.

After the removal of hemorrhoids or piles the patient often suffers considerably from swelling and throbbing pain. If but a portion of them have been removed the others may be temporarily much distended. Lint kept saturated with lead-water and laudanum, or some other soothing application, will frequently give great relief, as will the use of astringent and anodyne ointments prescribed by the surgeon.   A T-bandage and antiseptic pad will Dressings. need to be worn by the patient, and these will serve to hold the applications in place.

For the relief of hemorrhoids preparatory to Palliative treatment operation the application of cloths, wrung out in for hemor- rhoids. hot water, will serve to shrink them, and then, being anointed with vaseline or some simple oint- ment, they should be returned into the bowel.

Care to secure movements which are soft in con- After-care. sistency will be one of the chief objects in a nurse's attentions.   The measures already described in the use of oil enemata, combined with a laxative, are most effectual.   The patient's diet need not be restricted.   She may need to be confined to bed from ten days to two weeks, according to the severity of the case.

Lithotrity and lithotomy are operations for re- Operations for stone moval of stone from the bladder which are occa- in the bladder. sionally done through the urethra and vagina. The preparations for these, as for other pelvic operations, consist in free purgation and rest in bed for a day or two.   After the operation all efforts will be needed to allay irritation.

The patient must remain in bed and mild drinks After-man- agement. will probably need to be frequently administered,

16

as flaxseed-tea, barley water, soda water, milk, etc. The bedpan and urinal after lithotrity (crushing of the stone) should be used, and all fragments of stone kept for the doctor's inspection.

In lithotomy special provision will have to be made by means of pads for the protection of the bed from the dribbling of urine. Sometimes a tube is left in the wound for a few days, and the nurse will need to learn from the surgeon what he desires done to keep it free from obstruction. The nurse must make every effort to keep the patient quiet, clean, and dry. The hips and buttocks must be washed frequently and oiled, to prevent irritation from the constant escape of urine through the wound.

Symptoms to be reported.

Any appearance of blood in the urine must be reported to the surgeon, also any disposition to chilliness, profuse perspiration, tenderness about the lower part of the abdomen, etc.

Both these operations are done with the patient lying upon her back.

Operation for pelvic abscess.

The occurrence of abscess of the pelvis, which may point either externally or internally, sometimes demands the use of an apparatus known as the aspirator, which draws off the contents of the abscess by suction. A vacuum is produced in the bottle, as shown in the cut, by exhausting the air by means of the barrel and piston syringe. The

Management of aspirators.

return of air to the bottle being prevented by turning the small button on the side next the syringe
to close off communication there, and the valve on
the opposite side being opened by adjusting the
button on the needle-side properly, a suction power
is set up which draws out the contents of the

FIG. 67.

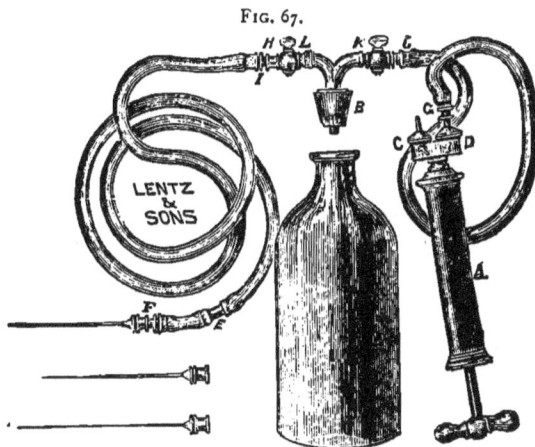

Aspirator and Needles.

abscess. A very thorough cleansing of the apparatus is necessary after such use.

The management of the case afterward will be After-care.
directed by the surgeon and will depend on the
location of the opening if one is made. If in the
vagina, antiseptic douches will be required. If an
external opening, a daily washing out of the

abscess cavity and re-dressing of the wound may
be necessary.

Dilatation
and curet-
ting of
uterus.

Operations for dilatation and curetting of the
uterus, or removal of polypi or retained placenta,
will need a similar preparation to that required for
all pelvic operations. Especial care must be given
to the employment of an antiseptic vaginal injec-

FIG. 68.

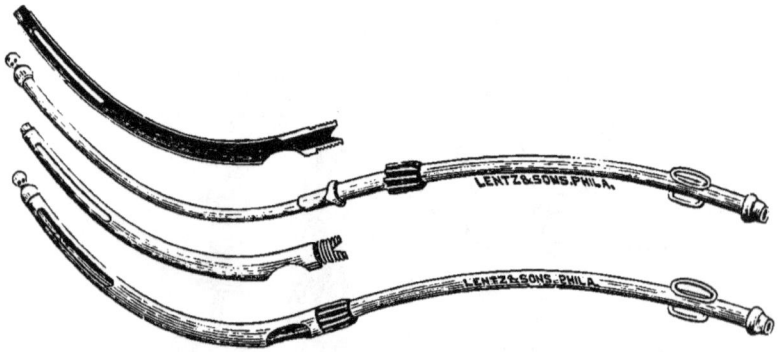

Intra-Uterine Return-Catheter.

tion just before operation. The patient will need
to be placed in the lithotomy position. During
the operation the uterus will probably need to be

Use of
intra-uter-
ine syringe.

washed out. For this purpose the intra-uterine
syringe, one form of which is shown in the cut,
may be employed. The lower figure shows the
instrument as it is put together for use, the upper
shows its separation into its three constituent parts.

It may be thus more thoroughly cleansed and rendered a safer instrument for use in different cases.

One end of a piece of flexible rubber tubing is slipped over the outer end of the catheter, and the other end over the nozzle connected with a fountain syringe. The solution used is contained in the rubber bag of the syringe, and, flowing down through the tubing and into one channel of the intra-uterine syringe, is carried into the uterus, being carried back through the other channel. Care must be taken in using these instruments to see that the return flow is free. If not, it may be possible that the instrument is clogged by a clot of blood or some shreds of tissue. It must then be removed and cleaned and reinserted. A thorough boiling or steaming of the instrument, after taking it apart, should follow its use.

Vaginal hysterectomy is an operation for the removal of the uterus through the vagina, and is most frequently done for cancer. *Vaginal hysterectomy.*

The patient is prepared as for perineal operation and placed in the lithotomy position upon the table, the limbs being held by the leg-holder. The after-management of the case will be dependent upon the methods preferred by the surgeon. If forceps are used to clamp the vessels, instead of ligatures being applied, they will extrude from the vagina, and the nurse will need to be careful in watching them to see that they do not loosen and drop off, and that there is no strain on them in the slight changes of position to which the patient may need to be subjected. In fact, the patient should be kept very quietly upon her back and all movements avoided until after the removal of the clamps, in two to three days. Quiet should be maintained after the removal of the clamps, to avoid the danger of secondary hemorrhage, until the surgeon declares all danger past. Antiseptic pads should be kept beneath the patient and frequently changed.

When ligatures are used a thick pad of iodoform-wool or gauze is laid over the vulva, after the tamponing of the vagina, and if a drainage-tube has been inserted in the vagina a sponge may be placed over its mouth. These dressings will be frequently inspected by the surgeon and changed if necessary. When the drainage-tube is used the pelvic cavity may have to be washed out should the temperature rise high or the discharge become offensive. Extreme care as to thorough asepsis will need to be practiced. The ligatures as a rule come away of themselves. If not, the surgeon may remove any sutures he may have introduced, and the remaining ligatures, at the end of two weeks. The patient will have to be placed on a table in the lithotomy position for this, and a Sims speculum used to depress the perineum.

As very especial danger of hemorrhage exists after this operation, extreme watchfulness will need to be exercised by the nurse in the care of a case of vaginal hysterectomy, and a frequent inspection should be made of the dressings to discover the amount and character of the discharge.

Operations on the breast may be done for the removal of tumors or cancer.   The arm-pit must be shaved and the breast made thoroughly clean by soap and water, followed by ether or turpentine for removing the grease from the skin, and then a thorough cleansing with bi-chloride solution, 1–1000.   The breast is then carefully enveloped in antiseptic dressings until the time for operation.   The patient is prepared as for other operations.   When it is near the time for operation the clothing may be removed from the side to be operated upon, but not from the other.   A thin sheet of rubber gossamer or, in a private house where this cannot be had, a folded sheet should go under the breast and arm of the affected side, being turned in over the clothing and fastened upon the opposite shoulder towards the front by a shield-pin.

The dressings should not be removed from the breast until the operator is ready to begin.   If there is any delay a shawl or blanket can be thrown

Amputation of the breast.

over the patient's shoulders until the surgeon is
ready.

Other pre-
parations.

The table for operation should be arranged as in
any other operation, except that the operating pad
should be placed at the upper part of the table,
under the affected shoulder. Sterilized towels may
be placed over the rubber-cloth protecting the pa-

The dress-
ings and
bandages.

tient's clothing. Special dressings will need to be
prepared for the case; thus, a large antiseptic pad
which shall reach front and back to the median line
of the body may be applied over the side of the
chest whence the breast was removed, and this
held in place by roller bandages firmly applied;
or, a straight bandage may hold the antiseptic
dressings in place, and a second one be used to
hold the arm firmly pinned down to the side.
These bandages may be prevented from slipping by
a strip of roller bandage fastened front and back
to their upper edge and passing over the shoulder.

After-care.

The patient should be kept perfectly quiet after
the operation. A little pillow 8 x 10 inches, of
down or feathers, may be slipped under the arm of
the affected side to support it and keep it from
dragging down. The nurse must watch especially

Watching
for hemor-
rhages.

for any tendency to hemorrhage. As the blood
will naturally run under the patient's back, owing
to her position, she must be gently lifted or rolled
towards the opposite side from time to time and the

back examined. Liquid food should be used for two or three days, unless the nurse is directed differently. Fresh dressings and bandages should be Redressing of wound. in readiness for the surgeon, as he may desire at any time to re-dress the wound. Should any discharge come through the dressings the surgeon should be at once notified of this, as it will be necessary in such case to change the dressings. The same antiseptic precautions should be observed in this re-dressing as in the original dressing of the wound.

Inflammation and abscess of the breast may Abscess of the breast. sometimes occur as a result of injury or of overdistention of the breast with milk during lactation. In preparing for the operation of lancing the breast the nurse will need to cleanse the breast thoroughly, and then wash it with an antiseptic solution and apply antiseptic dressings to keep it sterile until the time for operation. She should have in readiness a number of sterilized towels, a pus-pan or basin in which to catch the discharges, a tin basin containing carbolic solution for the instruments, an agate or china basin with a bi-chloride of mercury solution for the doctor's hands, soap, nail-brush, etc. The patient's clothing should be arranged as for amputation of the breast.

The instruments used will be the bistoury, straight or curved, and possibly a probe for subse-

quent packing of the cavity, with a strip of iodoform gauze.

Should the surgeon wish to use local anæsthesia
by means of ice and salt applied to the part, a bowl
containing a small quantity of salt and a piece of
smooth ice the size of a small fist, wrapped in a
towel, so that it can be thus held by the surgeon
while the application is made, should be provided.

Fig. 69.

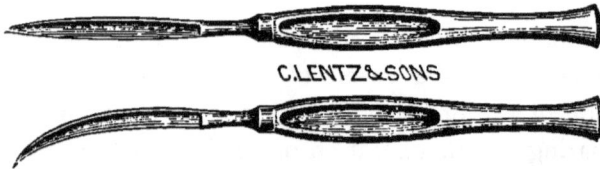

C.LENTZ&SONS

Bistouries, straight and curved.

Antiseptic dressings may be applied to the part
after lancing, or poultices may have, for a time,
to be kept up. In the latter case the poultice
should be made by mixing the meal with an antiseptic solution instead of plain water, in order
that thorough asepsis may be observed.

The abscess cavity will probably need to be
washed out daily with an antiseptic solution and
the breast re-dressed.

ANÆSTHESIA.

The administration of an anæsthetic, as ether or chloroform, does not often devolve upon the nurse; occasionally, however, the physician is obliged to call upon the nurse to aid him in this direction; it is therefore important that she should understand how to conduct the process. For general anæsthesia, ether is preferable to anything else because it is much the safest anæsthetic known. Chloroform is dangerous because of its direct action upon the heart

A patient should be prepared for etherization by taking nothing into the stomach for several hours previously. All the clothing should be loosened, false teeth should be removed, and the patient placed in a recumbent posture. The patient may be made to feel less nervous by one's placing the inhaler or towel over her mouth without any ether upon it and teaching her to draw deep breaths for a few seconds. A small handkerchief, loosely folded, may be saturated with about an ounce (two tablespoonfuls) of ether and held over the patient's mouth and nose, a dry towel being held over this to prevent the evaporation of the ether. The eyes may be covered by this towel. No talking should go on in the room, if possible, as the patient should be kept free from excitement. When inhalation has fully begun the ether cloth should not be removed from the patient's face, but more ether added by simply lifting the dry towel and adding the ether to the cloth beneath it. Should the patient stop breathing for a moment or the face become blue, the ether should be removed for a moment from the face. When a deep breath has been taken, the inhalation should be renewed. When during the stage of excitement the patient struggles and screams, the ether cloth should be held closely to the face, because giving her more air will simply make her noisier. The deep inspirations induced by crying and shouting often enable the inhalation to be more quickly effected. Retching is another symptom for which the ether should not be removed. If, however, the contents of the stomach are brought up into the throat and mouth, the etherization must be stopped until the mouth and throat have been cleared, or there will be danger of choking. The ether should be stopped for just as short a time as possible. When the mouth and throat become filled with an excessive secretion of mucus, it is also necessary to stop for a time and clear this away by carrying the finger into the mouth or by turning the patient over for a moment on her face or letting her head hang down for a moment over the operating table. When the patient breathes heavily, the muscles

are all relaxed, and on lifting the eyelid and touching the eye-ball the patient does not flinch, etherization is complete and the operator will be able to
begin his work.

The ether will after this need to be administered
in very small quantity. When the patient is
breathing heavily, making a snoring sound (ster-
torous breathing), the ether should not be pushed,
but the towel held some distance from the face.

Whenever ether is administered it should be
remembered that its vapor is inflammable, and so
heavy that it falls to the floor, so that any light, as
a candle or alcohol lamp, should be placed at a
distance from the operating table and on a higher
level.

When breathing ceases entirely and failure of
the heart seems to threaten, the patient's body
should be inverted and stimulants, as digitalis,
atropia, or aromatic spirit of ammonia, used hypo-
dermically. Every effort should be made to get
the patient to take a full breath. The tongue
should be drawn forward out of the mouth, the
cheeks and chest slapped with a towel wrung out
in cold water, artificial respiration may be resorted
to, or the use of electricity.

THE NURSE'S ARMAMENTARIUM.

A few words may be said in this connection of the nurse's armamentarium—the articles she will need to take with her to assist in the management of the cases she nurses.

A little pocket-case, containing a clinical thermometer, straight scissors, sharp-pointed and blunt-pointed, a pair of anatomical forceps, a probe, and a female catheter, is a convenience. An English or French male catheter is, also, often a necessity. Besides these the nurse will need a medicine glass, a feeder, and a nail-brush of her own; possibly a wall thermometer or bath thermometer might be added to the list, as it may save her delay in the use of douches, etc., as ordered, in case the family should not have anything of the kind.

Careful written reports should be kept of each case she nurses, and some blanks with the proper headings should be carried by her to each case. Thus properly equipped, she will be able to work more efficiently and satisfactorily to herself and to her patient.

FIG. 70.

DIAGRAM SHOWING NURSE'S REPORT. ABOUT ONE-FOURTH SIZE.

Patient's Name..   No. of page..................

Name of Nurse

DATE. | HOUR. | PULSE. | TEMP. | RESP. | FOOD. | MEDICINE AND TREATMENT. | URINE. | BOWEL MOVEMENTS. | REMARKS.

DIET FOR THE SICK.

LIQUID DIET.

BARLEY-WATER.

To one tablespoonful of ground barley add a pint of cold water; let it boil twenty minutes. Strain and keep in a cool place until used.

TOAST-MILK.

Toast two slices of baker's bread a dark brown, after drying thoroughly in the oven ; boil a pint of milk and pour it over the toast; strain and add either a little salt or sugar. Toast water is made in the same way, using water instead of milk.

FLAXSEED TEA.

To one quart of cold water add one tablespoonful of flaxseed; let simmer three or four hours ; strain ; add lemon juice and sugar to taste.

WINE WHEY.

When a pint of milk is brought just to a boil, pour in a gill of sherry wine ; let it again come to a boil ; when the whey separates, strain through gauze. It may be taken either warm or cold.

APPLE-WATER.

Pare, core, and cut into pieces a large, juicy apple; boil in a pint of water until the apple is tender enough to crush to a pulp; strain the liquor and sweeten to taste.

MILK-PUNCH.

Sweeten a glass three parts full of new milk to taste and add one or two tablespoonfuls of brandy or whiskey.

EGG-NOGG.

Stir well a heaping teaspoonful of sugar and the yolk of an egg in a glass and then add a table-spoonful of brandy or whiskey; fill the glass with new milk until it is three parts full, then stir into the mixture the white of the egg beaten to a stiff froth.

EGG-FLIP.

One egg, four teaspoonfuls of sugar, a glass three parts full of new milk; beat the egg and sugar together until light and stiff, then add to the milk.

TOAST-WINE.

One slice of well-browned toast, half a pint of boiling water, one teaspoonful of sugar, two tablespoonfuls of wine; put the toast into a pitcher, pour the boiling water over, and let stand until cold; then strain off the water and to it add the sugar and wine.

17

TODDY.

Half a glass of water, either hot or cold, half a teaspoonful of sugar, four teaspoonfuls of brandy or whiskey; dissolve the sugar in the water and add the brandy or whiskey.   If the juice of a lemon be added it makes lemon-toddy.

BEEF-TEA.

To one pint of cold water add one pound of chopped lean beef; let boil slowly four hours; strain and salt to taste.

QUICK BEEF-TEA.

One pound of chopped lean beef, half-a-pint of cold water, saltspoonful of salt; put the meat, water, and salt in a closely covered pan and boil gently ten minutes; stir well, strain, and remove the fat.

BEEF-BROTH.

One quart of cold water, one pound of lean, juicy beef; boil slowly for one hour; add a table-spoonful of rice, and salt to taste; when the rice is tender, strain the broth and serve with strips of dry toast.

Mutton broth is made in the same manner.

Chicken broth requires three pounds of chicken to two quarts of cold water.

OYSTER BROTH.

Cut one pint of oysters into small pieces, put them into a saucepan with half a pint of cold water ; boil gently ten minutes; skim, strain, and salt to taste. Serve hot with toasted crackers.

Clam broth is made in the same way.

EXPRESSED BEEF-JUICE.

Broil or pan lean beefsteak until it is heated through ; squeeze the juice out with either a beef press or a lemon squeezer ; strain through gauze to get the fat off. Before serving warm the juice in a small cup placed inside a cup of boiling water.

TO MAKE COFFEE.

Mix one tablespoonful of ground coffee with enough cold water to form a paste ; add one half-pint of boiling water ; boil a few minutes, then set it back on the range for a few moments to settle.

TO MAKE TEA.

Allow one small teaspoonful of tea to each cup ; add boiling water. Let the tea-pot stand at the side of the fire without boiling for a short time.

TO MAKE COCOA.

Mix one teaspoonful of cocoa with enough boiling water to form a paste ; add a cupful of boiling milk and serve immediately.

KOUMISS.

Fill a quart wine bottle up to the neck with pure milk ; add a quarter of a cake of compressed yeast and two tablespoonfuls of white sugar that have been dissolved in a little water over a hot fire. Tie the cork in the bottle securely and shake the bottle well. Place in a room of a temperature of from 50° to 90° F. for six hours, then in the ice-box over night.

SEMI-LIQUID DIET.

RICE-FLOUR GRUEL.

Mix two teaspoonfuls of rice flour with four tablespoonfuls of cold milk ; pour this into one pint of boiling milk, stirring all the time ; boil gently for fifteen minutes ; add sugar or salt to taste.

OATMEAL GRUEL.

Stir slowly one-half a cupful of rolled oats into one pint of boiling water; salt to taste and boil for twenty minutes.

FARINA GRUEL.

Sprinkle slowly one heaping tablespoonful of farina into one pint of boiling water, stirring all the time to prevent lumps ; boil for half an hour ; add salt to taste.

MEAL BALL.

Tie a pint of dry flour tightly in a piece of stout muslin and boil for nine hours; scrape off the outer crust, and the inside will be found to be a dry ball; grate this as needed, allowing one table-spoonful wet in cold milk to a pint of boiling milk; boil until smooth; add a salt spoonful of salt.

CORN-MEAL GRUEL.

Stir two even tablespoonfuls of corn meal into one pint of boiling water; boil gently for half an hour; salt to taste.

PEPTONIZED FOODS.

MILK PEPTONIZED BY HEAT.

Into a clean quart bottle put one measure (5 grs.) of Fairchild's Extractum Pancreatis, and one measure (15 grs.) of bicarbonate of soda, and a gill of cold water; shake; then add a pint of fresh, cold milk and shake the mixture again. Place the bottle in water about 110° to 115°, or so hot the whole hand can be held in it without discomfort for a minute. Keep the bottle there twenty minutes. At the end of that time put the bottle on ice to check further digestion and keep the milk from spoiling. Peptonized milk may be sweetened, flavored with grated nutmeg, or taken with mineral water. Put the mineral water first into the glass, then quickly pour in the peptonized milk, and drink during effervescence.

MILK PEPTONIZED BY COLD PROCESS.

Mix the peptonizing powder in cold water and cold milk as usual, and immediately place the bottle on ice, without subjecting it to the water bath or any heat. When needed pour out the required quantity and use in the same manner as ordinary milk.

SPECIALLY PEPTONIZED MILK FOR JELLIES, PUNCHES, ETC.

Mix the peptonizing powder (Extractum Pancreatis and bicarbonate of soda), cold water, and milk in a bottle, and place in a hot-water bath, as directed in recipe for peptonizing milk; let the bottle remain in the hot water for two hours, then pour into a sauce-pan and heat to boiling. This specially peptonized milk is now ready for jellies, etc. In peptonizing milk for recipes in which lemon juice or acid is to be used, it is necessary to carry the process to the point at which the milk will not curdle with acid. Hence the two hours' digestion. Do not fail to boil the milk immediately after the two hours in water bath, otherwise the milk will not set into a jelly, as the powder would digest the gelatine.

PEPTONIZED MILK JELLY.

First take about half a box of Nelson's gelatine, and set it aside to soak in a teacupful of cold water until needed; take one pint of specially peptonized milk heated hot; pare one lemon and one orange and throw the rinds into the specially prepared milk; squeeze the lemon and orange juice into a glass, strain, and mix it with two or three tablespoonfuls of wine or brandy; add to the milk, stirring well; strain through gauze, and when cooled to a sirupy consistency, so as to be almost ready to set, pour into moulds and set in a cool place. Do not pour the milk into the moulds until it is nearly cool, otherwise it will separate in setting.

PEPTONIZED MILK-PUNCH.

Take a glass about one-third full of fine crushed ice, pour on it a tablespoonful of brandy or whiskey, sweeten slightly and fill the glass with peptonized milk, stirring well.

MILK LEMONADE.

Take a glass one-third full of cracked ice; squeeze on it the juice of a lemon, sweeten to taste, and fill the glass with specially peptonized milk.

MILK-GRUEL.

Mix smoothly a heaping teaspoonful of wheat flour or arrowroot with half a pint of cold water; then heat, with constant stirring until it has boiled briskly, several minutes; mix with this hot gruel one pint of cold milk, and strain into a jar and immediately add one peptonizing powder; mix well. Let it stand in the hot water bath for 30 minutes, then put into a clean quart jar and place on ice.

PEPTONIZED BEEF.

One quarter of a pound of minced raw beef or beef and chicken mixed, or chicken alone; cold water one-half pint; cook over a slow fire, stirring constantly, until it has boiled a few minutes, then pour off the liquor and rub the meat to a paste, put it into a jar with one-half pint of cold water and the liquor poured from the meat, add four measures, or 20 grs., of Extractum Pancreatis, and one measure, or 15 grs., bicarbonate of soda; shake all well together and set aside in a warm place at about 110° or 115° F. for three hours, shaking occasionally, then boil quickly, strain and season. Be sure to boil the peptonized beef after three hours in a warm place, otherwise the digestion will progress until it is spoiled.

PEPTONIZED OYSTERS.

Half dozen large oysters with their juice and half pint of cold water; put into a saucepan and boil briskly for a few minutes; strain off the broth and set aside; mince the oysters and rub them to a paste; now put the oysters in a glass jar with the juice which has been set aside, and add three measures, or 15 grs., of Extractum Pancreatis, and one measure, or 15 grs., of bicarbonate of soda; let the jar stand in hot water, 115° F., for one and a half hours; pour into a saucepan, add half a pint of milk, and heat over the fire slowly to boiling point; strain, and season with salt and pepper. Heating the mixture *slowly* digests the milk sufficiently before the mixture boils. For a great majority of cases it will not be required to strain the peptonized liquor, for the portion of meat remaining undissolved will have been so softened and acted upon by the pancreatic extract that it will be in very fine particles, and diffused in an almost impalpable condition.

Farinaceous materials may also be used advantageously in the preparation of the peptonized soup by simply boiling a sufficient quantity of flour, arrowroot, rice, etc., with a half portion of the water used in the above recipe, and mixing all together, meat, gruel, Extractum Pancreatis, and soda. The pancreatine will at the same time digest both starch and meat. This has a more agreeable flavor than that made of meats alone. Jelly may also be made of peptonized beef. Beef-tea is peptonized in the same way as milk, using one pint of carefully strained cold beef-tea.

FARINACEOUS FOODS.

ARROWROOT CUSTARD.

Mix four tablespoonfuls of Bermuda arrowroot with one gill of cold milk, and pour it slowly into one pint of boiling milk, stirring all the time ; add two teaspoonfuls of sugar, a pinch of salt, and cook for fifteen minutes; flavor with nutmeg or ten drops of brandy ; pour it into a mould to cool. Serve with cream.

ARROWROOT WINE JELLY.

Mix two tablespoonfuls of Bermuda arrowroot with four tablespoonfuls of cold water and strain through gauze into half a pint of boiling water, stirring all the time; add two teaspoonfuls of sugar and simmer for five minutes, or until it looks perfectly clear ; remove from the fire, and stir in two tablespoonfuls of wine or brandy. Pour into a mould to cool.

ARROWROOT GRUEL.

Mix one tablespoonful of Bermuda arrowroot, a pinch of salt, and half a gill of cold water; stir into half a pint of boiling water and boil for fifteen minutes.

TAPIOCA JELLY.

Wash one tablespoonful of tapioca thoroughly and soak it in three gills of cold water over night, then simmer slowly until clear; add five teaspoonfuls of sugar and two teaspoonfuls of lemon juice and turn into a mould.

TAPIOCA CUSTARD.

One tablespoonful of tapioca soaked in two gills of cold water over night; boil until clear; put one gill of milk into a double kettle; beat together one egg, one teaspoonful of sugar, one half teaspoonful of corn-starch, and add to the gill of boiling milk; boil until about the consistency of cream; take from the fire and pour it into a bowl to cool; when cool stir in the stiff beaten white of an egg and the tapioca, and serve cold. Sago can be used in place of tapioca if desired.

FARINA CUSTARD.

Into two gills of boiling milk sprinkle one tablespoonful of farina, stirring all the time; boil for twenty minutes; then add the beaten yolk of one egg and one teaspoonful of sugar; let boil again and stir in the stiff beaten white of the egg; take from the fire, add a few drops of lemon or vanilla, if allowed, and turn out to cool.

EASILY PREPARED DESSERTS FOR CONVALESCENTS.

RICE SNOW.

Wash one tablespoonful of rice and boil until tender in a double boiler; add one tablespoonful of milk, one teaspoonful of sugar, a few drops of vanilla; while boiling stir in the stiff beaten white of one egg. Serve with cream either hot or cold.

` BREAD PUDDING.

Put one gill of dry bread crumbs into a small baking dish; pour two gills of boiling milk over them, cover close, and set aside to cool; beat together one heaping teaspoonful of sugar and one egg until very light, and stir into the bread and milk, which should be nearly cold; flavor with nutmeg and bake in a quick oven for twenty minutes. Serve hot with cream.

PLAIN RICE PUDDING.

Wash one-third of a cup of rice well; butter a pudding dish and stir in the rice, one pint of milk, and one tablespoonful of sugar; add a pinch of salt; grate nutmeg over it and bake for one and a half hours.

CORN-STARCH PUDDING.

Boil two gills of milk in a double kettle; dissolve one tablespoonful of corn-starch in a little cold milk and add to the boiling milk; boil for five minutes and then add the beaten yolk of one egg, one teaspoonful of vanilla, and one tablespoonful of sugar; turn into a buttered dish and bake in the oven for fifteen minutes; beat the white of the egg and a tablespoonful of pulverized sugar together until very light, spread over the pudding, and brown lightly in the oven. Instead of adding the yolk and baking the pudding, after adding the sugar and flavoring, stir in the well-beaten white of the egg, turn into a wet cup, and serve in a custard made of the yolk in this way: into one gill of boiling milk stir one half teaspoonful of corn-starch dissolved in one tablespoonful of milk; add the well-beaten yolk of the egg and one half teaspoonful of sugar; boil for five minutes; flavor with lemon or vanilla.

TIPSY PUDDING.

Half fill a small glass dish with stale sponge cake; mix together a tablespoonful of wine and tablespoonful of boiling water, and pour over the cake;

then fill the dish with custard made according to above recipe.

GERMAN TRIFLES.

In a small glass dish place a thin layer of sponge cake, then a layer of sliced orange, and pour custard over it. The white of the egg and one tablespoonful of pulverized sugar beaten very light may be piled on top when ready to serve.

APPLE FLOAT.

Stew and strain one large, tart apple; when cold add a tablespoonful of sugar and the well-beaten white of one egg. Serve as soon as made.

APPLE CUSTARD.

Stew and strain one large, tart apple; place over the fire, and while boiling add the beaten white of an egg and sugar to taste; place on ice, and before serving pile the beaten white and pulverized sugar on top of the custard. Serve with cream.

TAPIOCA AND FRUIT.

Wash a tablespoonful of tapioca and soak over night in three gills of cold water; then cook slowly until smooth and clear; add the juice of half a lemon, a teaspoonful of vanilla, and sugar to taste; place about a dozen large strawberries in a dish and pour the hot tapioca over them; then put on ice until ready to serve. Sliced peaches, raspberries, or bananas can be used in the same manner.

EGG JUNKET.

Beat one egg very light; add one teaspoonful of sugar, one half teaspoonful of vanilla, and two gills of lukewarm milk; put it into the dish it is to be served in and stir in one teaspoonful of rennet.

CHOCOLATE PUDDING.

Make a corn-starch pudding according to recipe given; when sufficiently boiled add one tablespoonful of grated chocolate; put the white of egg beaten stiff with one tablespoonful of pulverized sugar on top and brown slightly in oven.

WHIPPED CREAM.

Mix together two gills of rich cream, one half cup pulverized sugar, two tablespoonfuls sherry wine; put on ice for an hour, as cream whips much better if chilled; whip with an egg beater, and as the froth rises skim it off and lay it on a sieve to drain, returning the cream which drips away to be whipped over again. Place on the ice a short time before serving.

LEMON JELLY.

Cover one-third of a box of Nelson's gelatine with cold water and let it soak for fifteen minutes ; then add one cup of sugar, juice of one lemon, and two gills of boiling water; stir until the sugar is dissolved; strain through gauze and stand on ice to harden.

WINE JELLY.

Wine jelly is made the same, adding one gill of port or sherry wine instead of lemon juice.

ORANGE FLOAT.

Moisten one tablespoonful of corn-starch with a little cold water and stir it into two gills of boiling water, stirring constantly ; add one tablespoonful of sugar and the juice of one lemon; cut two oranges into small pieces, put into a dish, and pour the boiling corn-starch over them ; put on ice until needed.

TOUT FAIT.

Beat the yolk of an egg and a tablespoonful of sugar to a cream ; add one tablespoonful of milk and one of flour ; beat until smooth ; add the juice and rind of a lemon and the white of the egg beaten to a stiff froth ; turn into a buttered cup, dredge the top of the custard thickly with pulverized sugar, and bake in a quick oven for fifteen minutes.

STRAWBERRY SPONGE.

Cover one-half box of Nelson's gelatine with cold water and soak for half an hour, then pour over it one pint of boiling water; add one-half cup of sugar and stir until dissolved; add one-half pint of strawberry juice and strain into a basin; put this basin into a pan of cracked ice to stand until cold and stiff, stirring occasionally; then beat to a stiff froth, add the well-beaten whites of four eggs, beat until smooth; then place on the ice to harden.

CUP CUSTARD.

Beat one egg until light; add one teaspoonful of sugar; beat again; add one and a half gills of milk and nutmeg to taste and stir until the sugar is dissolved; pour into a buttered cup, place the cup in a pan of boiling water, and place in the oven. Bake until the custard sets; then set away to cool.

MISCELLANEOUS RECIPES.

BAKED POTATOES.

Select potatoes of same size; wash them well; bake in a clean, hot oven from 30 to 40 minutes, or until soft; break the skins to let the steam inside escape. Serve as soon as done.

CROUTONS.

Cut stale bread into half-inch slices; cut off the crust and cut into half-inch cubes; put them on a shallow pan and bake until brown. Use with beef-tea or broth.

BAKED APPLES.

Wipe the apples, remove the core, and put them in a pan; put sugar in the centre of each apple and enough water to cover the bottom of the pan; bake in a hot oven until soft, but not broken.

BAKED CRACKERS.

Split round crackers in halves, spread the inside with butter; put them buttered side up into a pan and brown in a hot oven.

BOILED POTATOES.

Select potatoes of nearly same size; wash them well; pare and cover with cold water; put them in a saucepan of boiling salted water (allowing one quart of water and one tablespoon even full of salt for six large potatoes); cook one-half hour or until soft; drain off every drop of water and place the saucepan uncovered at the back of the stove to let the steam escape. Serve hot.

RICE POTATO.

Mash the potatoes as soon as they are boiled, and press them through a colander into a hot dish.

MASHED POTATO.

To one pint of hot boiled potatoes add one table-spoonful of butter, one-half teaspoonful of salt, and enough hot milk to moisten; mash in the saucepan they were boiled in and beat with a fork until light and creamy; then turn into a hot dish.

POTATO CAKES.

Make cold, mashed potatoes into small, round cakes about one-half inch thick; put them into a baking pan, brush them over with milk, and bake in a hot oven until brown.

HARD-BOILED EGGS.

Cook them twenty minutes in water just bubbling; then the yolk is dry, mealy, and easily digested.

BOILED CUSTARD.

Beat one egg to a froth; add one tablespoonful of sugar and a little salt; mix well; add one cup of scalded milk and stir over boiling water until it thickens. Serve cold.

WATER TOAST.

Dip a slice of dry toast in salted boiling water; spread with butter and serve very hot.

MILK TOAST.

Dip a slice of dry toast in boiling milk which has a piece of butter dissolved in it.

BROILED STEAK.

Remove the bone and cut off the fat of a tender piece of steak; broil over a clear fire, turning the broiler every ten seconds; if it is to be rare, cook for four minutes. Serve on a hot plate with butter, salt, and pepper.

PANNED MUTTON CHOP.

Have the frying-pan hissing hot without any fat; take off the pink skin and outer fat of a chop, put it in the pan, and cook one minute; turn and sear on the other side, then cook more slowly until done—if rare, five minutes will be long enough; when nearly done, sprinkle a little salt on each side. Drain on paper and serve very hot on a very hot plate without a drop of grease.

BAKED APPLE SAUCE.

Fill a small baking dish with apples, pared, cored, and quartered; allow one-half cup of sugar for one quart of apples, also one cup of water; bake, covered, in a slow oven until clear.

STEWED PRUNES.

Wash one pound of prunes and soak them for one hour before cooking; put them in a granite pan and cover with boiling water; simmer until swollen and tender, then add one tablespoonful of sugar; cook ten minutes longer and set away to cool.

STEWED OYSTERS.

Put a pint of oysters in a pan and heat until the edges curl; then add one cup of boiling milk that is salted to taste; butter and pepper may be added if allowed.

STEWED CRANBERRIES.

Wash and pick one cup of cranberries; put them in a saucepan and sprinkle one-half cup of sugar over them; pour out one-fourth cup of water, and after they begin to boil cook them for ten minutes, closely covered; do not stir them. They will jelly when cold and are much nicer than when strained.

STEAMED RHUBARB.

Wash enough rhubarb cut into inch pieces to fill a cup; put it into a double boiler; sprinkle one-half cup of sugar over it and steam until soft. Do not stir it.

BROILED FISH.

To broil mackerel, white fish, small blue fish, trout, small cod, shad, or any other thin fish, split them down the back and remove the head and tail. Sometimes it is well to remove the backbone also. To broil halibut, salmon, and other thick fish, cut them into inch-thick slices across the back-bone and remove the bone and skin. Oily fish need only salt and pepper, but dry white fish should be spread with soft butter before broiling.

Grease a double wire broiler with lard or butter; put the thickest edge of the fish next the middle of the broiler; broil the flesh side first until it is brown, lifting it up often that it may not burn; cook the other side enough just to crisp the skin—the time will vary with the thickness of the fish; the flesh when done should look firm and white and separate easily from the bone; loosen the fish from each side of the broiler, open the broiler and slide off the fish, or hold a plate over the skin side of the fish and invert plate and broiler together; season with pepper and salt.

SAUCE FOR FISH.

Put a pint of water in a saucepan; add half-tea-spoonful of salt; mix one-half cup of butter and two tablespoonfuls of flour together; when perfectly smooth, add to the boiling water, stir rapidly until it thickens—if not free from lumps strain the sauce. To make egg sauce, add to the drawn butter two hard-boiled eggs, sliced, or one tablespoonful of finely chopped parsley may be added.

WEIGHTS AND MEASURES.

FLUID MEASURE.

℥ 60	=	f ℨ j
f ℨ viij	=	f ℥ j
f ℥ xvj	=	Oj
Oviij	=	Cj.

APOTHECARIES' MEASURE.

gr.xx	=	℈ j
℈ iij	=	ℨ j
ℨ viij	=	℥ j
℥ xij	=	lb.j.

DOMESTIC MEASURES.

1 teaspoonful, about one fluidrachm	=	f ℨ j
1 tablespoonful, " ½ fluidounce	=	f ℥ ss
1 wineglassful, " 2 fluidounces	=	f ℥ ij
1 teacupful, " 4 fluidounces	=	f ℥ iv
1 coffeecupful, " 8 fluidounces	=	f ℥ viij.

INDEX.

281

A CATALOGUE

OF

BOOKS FOR STUDENTS.

INCLUDING THE

? QUIZ-COMPENDS ?

CONTENTS.

PUBLISHED BY

P. BLAKISTON, SON & CO.,

Medical Booksellers, Importers and Publishers.

LARGE STOCK OF ALL STUDENTS' BOOKS, AT

THE LOWEST PRICES.

1012 Walnut Street, Philadelphia.

₊ For sale by all Booksellers, or any book will be sent by mail, postpaid, upon receipt of price. Catalogues of books on all branches of Medicine, Dentistry, Pharmacy, etc., supplied upon application.

☞ Gould's New Medical Dictionary Just Ready. *See page 16.*

A NEW SERIES OF
STUDENTS' MANUALS

On the various Branches of Medicine and Surgery.

Can be used by Students of any College.

Price of each, Handsome Cloth, $3.00. Full Leather, $3.50.

The object of this series is to furnish good manuals for the medical student, that will strike the medium between the compend on one hand and the prolix text-book on the other—to contain all that is necessary for the student, without embarrassing him with a flood of theory and involved statements. They have been prepared by well-known men, who have had large experience as teachers and writers, and who are, therefore, well informed as to the needs of the student.

Their mechanical execution is of the best—good type and paper, handsomely illustrated whenever illustrations are of use, and strongly bound in uniform style.

Each book is sold separately at a remarkably low price, and the immediate success of several of the volumes shows that the series has met with popular favor.

No. 1. SURGERY. 236 Illustrations.

A Manual of the Practice of Surgery. By Wм. J. WALSHAM, M.D., Asst. Surg. to, and Demonstrator of Surg. in, St. Bartholomew's Hospital, London, etc. 236 Illustrations.

Presents the introductory facts in Surgery in clear, precise language, and contains all the latest advances in Pathology, Antiseptics, etc.

" It aims to occupy a position midway between the pretentious manual and the cumbersome System of Surgery, and its general character may be summed up in one word—practical."—*The Medical Bulletin.*

" Walsham, besides being an excellent surgeon, is a teacher in its best sense, and having had very great experience in the preparation of candidates for examination, and their subsequent professional career, may be relied upon to have carried out his work successfully. Without following out in detail his arrangement, which is excellent, we can at once say that his book is an embodiment of modern ideas neatly strung together, with an amount of careful organization well suited to the candidate, and, indeed, to the practitioner."—*British Medical Journal.*

Price of each Book, Cloth, $3.00; Leather, $3.50.

No. 2. DISEASES OF WOMEN. 150 Illus.
NEW EDITION.

The Diseases of Women. Including Diseases of the Bladder and Urethra. By DR. F. WINCKEL, Professor of Gynæcology and Director of the Royal University Clinic for Women, in Munich. Second Edition. Revised and Edited by Theophilus Parvin, M.D., Professor of Obstetrics and Diseases of Women and Children in Jefferson Medical College.   150 Engravings, most of which are original.

" The book will be a valuable one to physicians, and a safe and satisfactory one to put into the hands of students. It is issued in a neat and attractive form, and at a very reasonable price."—*Boston Medical and Surgical Journal.*

No. 3. OBSTETRICS. 227 Illustrations.

A Manual of Midwifery. By ALFRED LEWIS GALABIN, M.A., M.D., Obstetric Physician and Lecturer on Midwifery and the Diseases of Women at Guy's Hospital, London; Examiner in Midwifery to the Conjoint Examining Board of England, etc. With 227 Illus.

" This manual is one we can strongly recommend to all who desire to study the science as well as the practice of midwifery. Students at the present time not only are expected to know the principles of diagnosis, and the treatment of the various emergencies and complications that occur in the practice of midwifery, but find that the tendency is for examiners to ask more questions relating to the science of the subject than was the custom a few years ago. * * * The general standard of the manual is high ; and wherever the science and practice of midwifery are well taught it will be regarded as one of the most important text-books on the subject."—*London Practitioner.*

No. 4. PHYSIOLOGY. Fifth Edition.
321 ILLUSTRATIONS AND A GLOSSARY.

A Manual of Physiology. By GERALD F. YEO, M.D., F.R.C.S., Professor of Physiology in King's College, London.   321 Illustrations and a Glossary of Terms. Fifth American from last English Edition, revised and improved. 758 pages.

This volume was specially prepared to furnish students with a new text-book of Physiology, elementary so far as to avoid theories which have not borne the test of time and such details of methods as are unnecessary for students in our medical colleges.

" The brief examination I have given it was so favorable that I placed it in the list of text-books recommended in the circular of the University Medical College."—*Prof. Lewis A. Stimson,* M.D., *37 East 33d Street, New York.*

Price of each Book, Cloth, $3.00 ; Leather, $3.50.

No. 5. DISEASES OF CHILDREN.

SECOND EDITION.

A Manual. By J. F. GOODHART, M.D., Phys. to the Evelina Hospital for Children; Asst. Phys. to Guy's Hospital, London. Second American Edition. Edited and Rearranged by LOUIS STARR, M.D., Clinical Prof. of Dis. of Children in the Hospital of the Univ. of Pennsylvania, and Physician to the Children's Hospital, Phila. Containing many new Prescriptions, a list of over 50 Formulæ, conforming to the U. S. Pharmacopœia, and Directions for making Artificial Human Milk, for the Artificial Digestion of Milk, etc.   Illus.

"The merits of the book are many. Aside from the praiseworthy work of the printer and binder, which gives us a print and page that delights the eye, there is the added charm of a style of writing that is not wearisome, that makes its statements clearly and forcibly, and that knows when to stop when it has said enough. The insertion of typical temperature charts certainly enhances the value of the book. It is rare, too, to find in any text-book so many topics treated of. All the rarer and out-of-the-way diseases are given consideration. This we commend. It makes the work valuable."—*Archives of Pedriatics, July, 1890.*

"The author has avoided the not uncommon error of writing a book on general medicine and labeling it 'Diseases of Children,' but has steadily kept in view the diseases which seemed to be incidental to childhood, or such points in disease as appear to be so peculiar to or pronounced in children as to justify insistence upon them. * * * A safe and reliable guide, and in many ways admirably adapted to the wants of the student and practitioner."— *American Journal of Medical Science.*

"Thoroughly individual, original and earnest, the work evidently of a close observer and an independent thinker, this book, though small, as a handbook or compendium is by no means made up of bare outlines or standard facts."—*The Therapeutic Gazette.*

"As it is said of some men, so it might be said of some books, that they are 'born to greatness.' This new volume has, we believe, a mission, particularly in the hands of the younger members of the profession. In these days of prolixity in medical literature, it is refreshing to meet with an author who knows both what to say and when he has said it. The work of Dr. Goodhart (admirably conformed, by Dr. Starr, to meet American requirements) is the nearest approach to clinical teaching without the actual presence of clinical material that we have yet seen."—*New York Medical Record.*

Price of each Book, Cloth, $3.00; Leather, $3.50.

No. 6. PRACTICAL THERAPEUTICS.

FOURTH EDITION, WITH AN INDEX OF DISEASES.

Practical Therapeutics, considered with reference to Articles of the Materia Medica. Containing, also, an Index of Diseases, with a list of the Medicines applicable as Remedies. By EDWARD JOHN WARING, M.D., F.R.C.P. Fourth Edition. Rewritten and Revised by DUDLEY W. BUXTON, M.D., Asst. to the Prof. of Medicine at University College Hospital.

" We wish a copy could be put in the hands of every Student or Practitioner in the country. In our estimation, it is the best book of the kind ever written."—*N. Y. Medical Journal.*

" Dr. Waring's Therapeutics has long been known as one of the most thorough and valuable of medical works. The amount of actual intellectual labor it represents is immense. . . . An index of diseases, with the remedies appropriate for their treatment, closes the volume."—*Boston Medical and Surgical Reporter.*

" The plan of this work is an admirable one, and one well calculated to meet the wants of busy practitioners. There is a remarkable amount of information, accompanied with judicious comments, imparted in a concise yet agreeable style."—*Medical Record.*

No. 7. MEDICAL JURISPRUDENCE AND TOXICOLOGY.

THIRD REVISED EDITION.

By JOHN J. REESE, M.D., Professor of Medical Jurisprudence and Toxicology in the University of Pennsylvania; President of the Medical Jurisprudence Society of Phila.; Third Edition, Revised and Enlarged.

"This admirable text-book."—*Amer. Jour. of Med. Sciences.*

" We lay this volume aside, after a careful perusal of its pages, with the profound impression that it should be in the hands of every doctor and lawyer. It fully meets the wants of all students. . . . . He has succeeded in admirably condensing into a handy volume all the essential points."—*Cincinnati Lancet and Clinic.*

" The book before us will, we think, be found to answer the expectations of the student or practitioner seeking a manual of jurisprudence, and the call for a second edition is a flattering testimony to the value of the author's present effort. The medical portion of this volume seems to be uniformly excellent, leaving little for adverse criticism. The information on the subject matter treated has been carefully compiled, in accordance with recent knowledge. The toxicological portion appears specially excellent. Of that portion of the work treating of the legal relations of the practitioner and medical witness, we can express a generally favorable verdict."—*Physician and Surgeon, Ann Arbor, Mich.*

Price of each Book, Cloth, $3,00; Leather, $3.50.

ANATOMY.

Macalister's Human Anatomy. 816 Illustrations. A new Text-book for Students and Practitioners, Systematic and Topographical, including the Embryology, Histology and Morphology of Man. With special reference to the requirements of Practical Surgery and Medicine. With 816 Illustrations, 400 of which are original. Octavo.   Cloth, 7.50 ; Leather, 8.50

Ballou's Veterinary Anatomy and Physiology. Illustrated. By Wm. R. Ballou, M.D., Professor of Equine Anatomy at New York College of Veterinary Surgeons. 29 graphic Illustrations. 12mo.   Cloth, 1.00 ; Interleaved for notes, 1.25

Holden's Anatomy. A manual of Dissection of the Human Body. Fifth Edition. Enlarged, with Marginal References and over 200 Illustrations. Octavo.

   Bound in Oilcloth, for the Dissecting Room, $4.50.

   " No student of Anatomy can take up this book without being pleased and instructed. Its Diagrams are original, striking and suggestive, giving more at a glance than pages of text description. * * * The text matches the illustrations in directness of practical application and clearness of detail."—*New York Medical Record.*

Holden's Human Osteology. Comprising a Description of the Bones, with Colored Delineations of the Attachments of the Muscles. The General and Microscopical Structure of Bone and its Development. With Lithographic Plates and Numerous Illustrations. Seventh Edition. 8vo.   Cloth, 6.00

Holden's Landmarks, Medical and Surgical. 4th ed. Clo., 1.25

Heath's Practical Anatomy. Sixth London Edition. 24 Colored Plates, and nearly 300 other Illustrations.   Cloth, 5.00

Potter's Compend of Anatomy. Fifth Edition. Enlarged. 16 Lithographic Plates. 117 Illustrations. *See Page 14.*
   Cloth, 1.00 ; Interleaved for Notes, 1.25

CHEMISTRY.

Bartley's Medical Chemistry. Second Edition. A text-book prepared specially for Medical, Pharmaceutical and Dental Students. With 50 Illustrations, Plate of Absorption Spectra and Glossary of Chemical Terms. Revised and Enlarged. Cloth, 2.50

Trimble. Practical and Analytical Chemistry. A Course in Chemical Analysis, by Henry Trimble, Prof. of Analytical Chemistry in the Phila. College of Pharmacy. Illustrated. Third Edition. 8vo.   Cloth, 1.50

   ☞ *See pages 2 to 5 for list of Students' Manuals.*

Chemistry:—Continued.

Bloxam's Chemistry, Inorganic and Organic, with Experiments. Seventh Edition. Enlarged and Rewritten. 281 Illustrations.
Cloth, 4.50; Leather, 5.50

Richter's Inorganic Chemistry. A text-book for Students. Third American, from Fifth German Edition. Translated by Prof. Edgar F. Smith, PH.D. 89 Wood Engravings and Colored Plate of Spectra. Cloth, 2.00

Richter's Organic Chemistry, or Chemistry of the Carbon Compounds. Illustrated. Second Edition. Cloth, 4.50

Symonds. Manual of Chemistry, for the special use of Medical Students. By BRANDRETH SYMONDS, A.M., M.D., Asst. Physician Roosevelt Hospital, Out-Patient Department; Attending Physician Northwestern Dispensary, New York. 12mo.
Cloth, 2.00; Interleaved for Notes, 2.40

Leffmann's Compend of Chemistry. Inorganic and Organic. Including Urinary Analysis. Third Edition. Revised.
Cloth, 1.00; Interleaved for Notes, 1.25

Leffmann and Beam. Progressive Exercises in Practical Chemistry. 12mo. Illustrated. Cloth, 1.00

Muter. Practical and Analytical Chemistry. Fourth Edition. Revised, to meet the requirements of American Medical Colleges, by Prof. C. C. Hamilton. Illustrated. Cloth, 2.00

Holland. The Urine, Common Poisons, and Milk Analysis, Chemical and Microscopical. For Laboratory Use. Fourth Edition, Enlarged. Illustrated. Cloth, 1.00

Van Nüys. Urine Analysis. Illus. Cloth, 2.00

Wolff's Applied Medical Chemistry. By Lawrence Wolff, M.D., Dem. of Chemistry in Jefferson Medical College. Clo., 1.00

CHILDREN.

Goodhart and Starr. The Diseases of Children. Second Edition. By J. F. Goodhart, M.D., Physician to the Evelina Hospital for Children; Assistant Physician to Guy's Hospital, London. Revised and Edited by Louis Starr, M.D., Clinical Professor of Diseases of Children in the Hospital of the University of Pennsylvania; Physician to the Children's Hospital, Philadelphia. Containing many Prescriptions and Formulæ, conforming to the U. S. Pharmacopœia, Directions for making Artificial Human Milk, for the Artificial Digestion of Milk, etc. Illustrated. Cloth, 3.00; Leather, 3.50

Hatfield. Diseases of Children. By M. P. Hatfield, M.D., Professor of Diseases of Children, Chicago Medical College. Colored Plate. 12mo. Cloth, 1.00; Interleaved, 1.25

☞ *See pages 14 and 15 for list of ? Quiz-Compends ?*

Children:—Continued.

Starr. **Diseases of the Digestive Organs in Infancy and Childhood.** With chapters on the Investigation of Disease, and on the General Management of Children. By Louis Starr, M.D., Clinical Professor of Diseases of Children in the University of Pennsylvania. Illus. Second Edition.   Cloth, 2.25

DENTISTRY.

Fillebrown. **Operative Dentistry.** 330 Illus.   Cloth, 2.50

Flagg's Plastics and Plastic Filling. 4th Ed.   Cloth, 4.00

Gorgas. **Dental Medicine.** A Manual of Materia Medica and Therapeutics. Fourth Edition.   Cloth, 3.50

Harris. **Principles and Practice of Dentistry.** Including Anatomy, Physiology, Pathology, Therapeutics, Dental Surgery and Mechanism. Twelfth Edition. Revised and enlarged by Professor Gorgas. 1028 Illustrations. Cloth, 7.00 ; Leather, 8.00

Richardson's Mechanical Dentistry. Fifth Edition. 569 Illustrations. 8vo.   Cloth, 4.50; Leather, 5.50

Sewill. **Dental Surgery.** 200 Illustrations. 3d Ed. Clo., 3.00

Taft's Operative Dentistry. Dental Students and Practitioners. Fourth Edition. 100 Illustrations.   Cloth, 4.25 ; Leather, 5.00

Talbot. **Irregularities of the Teeth,** and their Treatment. Illustrated. 8vo. Second Edition.   Cloth, 3.00

Tomes' Dental Anatomy. Third Ed. 191 Illus. Cloth, 4.00

Tomes' Dental Surgery. 3d Edition. Revised. 292 Illus. 772 Pages.   Cloth, 5.00

Warren. **Compend of Dental Pathology and Dental Medicine.** Illustrated.   Cloth, 1.00 ; Interleaved, 1.25

DICTIONARIES.

Gould's New Medical Dictionary. Containing the Definition and Pronunciation of all words in Medicine, with many useful Tables etc. ½ Dark Leather, 3.25 ; ½ Mor., Thumb Index 4.25

Harris' Dictionary of Dentistry. Fifth Edition. Completely revised and brought up to date by Prof. Gorgas.
         Cloth, 5.00 ; Leather, 6.00

Cleaveland's Pronouncing Pocket Medical Lexicon. 31st Edition. Giving correct Pronunciation and Definition. Very small pocket size. Cloth, red edges .75 ; pocket-book style, 1.00

Longley's Pocket Dictionary. The Student's Medical Lexicon, giving Definition and Pronunciation of all Terms used in Medicine, with an Appendix giving Poisons and Their Antidotes, Abbreviations used in Prescriptions, Metric Scale of Doses, etc. 24mo.   Cloth, 1.00 ; pocket-book style, 1.25

☞ See pages 2 to 5 for list of Students' Manuals.

EYE.

Hartridge on Refraction. 4th Edition.   Cloth, 2.00

Hartridge on the Ophthalmoscope.   *Nearly Ready.*

Meyer. Diseases of the Eye. A complete Manual for Students and Physicians. 270 Illustrations and two Colored Plates. 8vo.   Cloth, 4.50; Leather, 5.50

Swanzy. Diseases of the Eye and their Treatment. 158 Illustrations. Third Edition.   Cloth, 3 00

Fox and Gould. Compend of Diseases of the Eye and Refraction. 2d Ed. Enlarged. 71 Illus. 39 Formulæ.
                    Cloth, 1.00; Interleaved for Notes, 1.25

ELECTRICITY.

Bigelow. Plain Talks on Medical Electricity and Batteries. Illustrated. With a Glossary of Electrical Terms.   Cloth, 1.00

Mason's Compend of Medical and Surgical Electricity. With numerous Illustrations. 12mo.   Cloth, 1.00

HYGIENE.

Parkes' (Ed. A.) Practical Hygiene. Seventh Edition, enlarged. Illustrated. 8vo.   Cloth, 4.50

Parkes' (L. C.) Manual of Hygiene and Public Health. Second Edition. 12mo.   Cloth, 2.50

Wilson's Handbook of Hygiene and Sanitary Science. Seventh Edition. Revised and Illustrated.   *In Press.*

MATERIA MEDICA AND THERAPEUTICS.

Potter's Compend of Materia Medica, Therapeutics and Prescription Writing. Fifth Edition, revised and improved. *See Page 15.*   Cloth, 1.00; Interleaved for Notes, 1.25

Biddle's Materia Medica. Eleventh Edition. By the late John B. Biddle, M.D., Prof. of Materia Medica in Jefferson College, Philadelphia. Revised by Clement Biddle, M.D., and Henry Morris, M.D. 8vo., illustrated. Cloth, 4.25; Leather, 5.00

Potter. Handbook of Materia Medica, Pharmacy and Therapeutics. Including Action of Medicines, Special Therapeutics, Pharmacology, etc. By Saml. O. L. Potter, M.D., M.R.C.P. (Lond.), Professor of the Practice of Medicine in Cooper Medical College, San Francisco. Third Edition. 8vo.
                              Cloth, 4.00; Leather, 5.00

Waring. Therapeutics. With an Index of Diseases and Remedies. 4th Edition. Revised. Cloth, 3.00; Leather, 3.50

☞ *See pages 14 and 15 for list of ? Quiz-Compends ?*

MEDICAL JURISPRUDENCE.

Reese. A Text-book of Medical Jurisprudence and Toxicology. By John J. Reese, M.D., Professor of Medical Jurisprudence and Toxicology in the Medical Department of the University of Pennsylvania; President of the Medical Jurisprudence Society of Philadelphia; Physician to St. Joseph's Hospital; Corresponding Member of The New York Medico-legal Society. Third Edition.   Cloth, 3.00; Leather, 3.50

OBSTETRICS AND GYNÆCOLOGY.

Davis. A Manual of Obstetrics. Colored Plates, and 150 other Illustrations.   *Ready in October, 1891.*

Byford. Diseases of Women. The Practice of Medicine and Surgery, as applied to the Diseases and Accidents Incident to Women. By W. H. Byford, A.M., M.D., Professor of Gynæcology in Rush Medical College and of Obstetrics in the Woman's Medical College, etc., and Henry T. Byford, M.D., Surgeon to the Woman's Hospital of Chicago. Fourth Edition. Revised and Enlarged. 306 Illustrations, over 100 of which are original. Octavo. 832 pages.   Cloth, 5.00; Leather, 6.00

Cazeaux and Tarnier's Midwifery. With Appendix, by Mundé. The Theory and Practice of Obstetrics; including the Diseases of Pregnancy and Parturition, Obstetrical Operations, etc. Eighth American, from the Eighth French and First Italian Edition. Edited by Robert J. Hess, M.D., Physician to the Northern Dispensary, Philadelphia, with an appendix by Paul F. Mundé, M.D., Professor of Gynæcology at the N. Y. Polyclinic. Illustrated by Chromo-Lithographs, and other Full-page Plates, seven of which are beautifully colored, and numerous Wood Engravings. One Vol., 8vo.   Cloth, 5.00; Leather, 6.00

Lewers' Diseases of Women. A Practical Text-Book. 139 Illustrations. Second Edition.   Cloth, 2.50

Parvin's Winckel's Diseases of Women. Second Edition. Including a Section on Diseases of the Bladder and Urethra. 150 Illus. Revised. *See page 3.*   Cloth, 3.00; Leather, 3.50

Morris. Compend of Gynæcology. Illustrated.   Cloth, 1.00

Winckel's Obstetrics. A Text-book on Midwifery, including the Diseases of Childbed. By Dr. F. Winckel, Professor of Gynæcology, and Director of the Royal University Clinic for Women, in Munich. Authorized Translation, by J. Clifton Edgar, M.D., Lecturer on Obstetrics, University Medical College, New York, with nearly 200 handsome illustrations, the majority of which are original. 8vo. Cloth, 6.00; Leather, 7.00

Landis' Compend of Obstetrics. Illustrated. 4th edition, enlarged.   Cloth, 1.00; Interleaved for Notes, 1.25

Galabin's Midwifery. By A. Lewis Galabin, M.D., F.R.C.P. 227 Illustrations. *See page 3.*   Cloth, 3.00; Leather, 3.50

Rigby's Obstetric Memoranda. 4th Edition.   Cloth, .50

☞ *See pages 2 to 5 for list of New Manuals.*

PATHOLOGY. HISTOLOGY. BIOLOGY.

Bowlby. Surgical Pathology and Morbid Anatomy, for Students. 135 Illustrations. 12mo. Cloth, 2.00

Davis' Elementary Biology. Illustrated. Cloth, 4.00

Gilliam's Essentials of Pathology. A Handbook for Students. 47 Illustrations. 12mo. Cloth, 2.00

****** The object of this book is to unfold to the beginner the fundamentals of pathology in a plain, practical way, and by bringing them within easy comprehension to increase his interest in the study of the subject.

Gibbes' Practical Histology and Pathology. Third Edition. Enlarged. 12mo. Cloth, 1.75

Virchow's Post-Mortem Examinations. 3d Ed. Cloth, 1.00

PHYSICAL DIAGNOSIS.

Fenwick. Student's Guide to Physical Diagnosis. 7th Edition. 117 Illustrations. 12mo. Cloth, 2.25

Tyson's Physical Diagnosis. Illustrated.
To be ready, October, 1891.

PHYSIOLOGY.

Yeo's Physiology. Fifth Edition. The most Popular Students' Book. By Gerald F. Yeo, M.D., F.R.C.S., Professor of Physiology in King's College, London. Small Octavo. 758 pages. 321 carefully printed Illustrations. With a Full Glossary and Index. *See Page 3.* Cloth, 3.00; Leather, 3.50

Brubaker's Compend of Physiology. Illustrated. Sixth Edition. Cloth, 1.00; Interleaved for Notes, 1.25

Stirling. Practical Physiology, including Chemical and Experimental Physiology. 142 Illustrations. Cloth, 2.25

Kirke's Physiology. New 12th Ed. Thoroughly Revised and Enlarged. 502 Illustrations. Cloth, 4.00; Leather, 5.00

Landois' Human Physiology. Including Histology and Microscopical Anatomy, and with special reference to Practical Medicine. Third Edition. Translated and Edited by Prof. Stirling. 692 Illustrations. Cloth, 6.50; Leather, 7.50

"With this Text-book at his command, no student could fail in his examination."—*Lancet.*

Sanderson's Physiological Laboratory. Being Practical Exercises for the Student. 350 Illustrations. 8vo. Cloth, 5.00

PRACTICE.

Taylor. Practice of Medicine. A Manual. By Frederick Taylor, M.D., Physician to, and Lecturer on Medicine at, Guy's Hospital, London; Physician to Evelina Hospital for Sick Children, and Examiner in Materia Medica and Pharmaceutical Chemistry, University of London. Cloth, 4.00; Leather, 5.00

☞ *See pages 14 and 15 for list of ? Quiz-Compends ?*

Practice:—Continued.

Roberts' Practice. New Revised Edition. A Handbook of the Theory and Practice of Medicine. By Frederick T. Roberts, M.D.; M.R.C.P., Professor of Clinical Medicine and Therapeutics in University College Hospital, London. Seventh Edition. Octavo.   Cloth, 5.50; Sheep, 6.50

Hughes. Compend of the Practice of Medicine. 4th Edition. Two parts, each, Cloth, 1.00; Interleaved for Notes, 1.25

PART I.—Continued, Eruptive and Periodical Fevers, Diseases of the Stomach, Intestines, Peritoneum, Biliary Passages, Liver, Kidneys, etc., and General Diseases, etc.

PART II.—Diseases of the Respiratory System, Circulatory System and Nervous System; Diseases of the Blood, etc.

Physicians' Edition. Fourth Edition. Including a Section on Skin Diseases. With Index. 1 vol. Full Morocco, Gilt, 2.50

From John A. Robinson, M.D., Assistant to Chair of Clinical Medicine, now Lecturer on Materia Medica, Rush Medical College, Chicago.

"Meets with my hearty approbation as a substitute for the ordinary note books almost universally used by medical students. It is concise, accurate, well arranged and lucid, . . . just the thing for students to use while studying physical diagnosis and the more practical departments of medicine."

PRESCRIPTION BOOKS.

Wythe's Dose and Symptom Book. Containing the Doses and Uses of all the principal Articles of the Materia Medica, etc. Seventeenth Edition. Completely Revised and Rewritten. *Just Ready.* 32mo.   Cloth, 1.00; Pocket-book style, 1.25

Pereira's Physician's Prescription Book. Containing Lists of Terms, Phrases, Contractions and Abbreviations used in Prescriptions Explanatory Notes, Grammatical Construction of Prescriptions, etc., etc. By Professor Jonathan Pereira, M.D. Sixteenth Edition. 32mo. Cloth, 1.00; Pocket-book style, 1.25

PHARMACY.

Stewart's Compend of Pharmacy. Based upon Remington's Text-Book of Pharmacy. Third Edition, Revised. With new Tables, Index, Etc.   Cloth, 1.00; Interleaved for Notes, 1.25

Robinson. Latin Grammar of Pharmacy and Medicine. By H. D. Robinson, PH.D., Professor of Latin Language and Literature, University of Kansas, Lawrence. With an Introduction by L. E. Sayre, PH.G., Professor of Pharmacy in, and Dean of, the Dept. of Pharmacy, University of Kansas. 12mo.
Cloth, 2.00

SKIN DISEASES.

Anderson, (McCall) Skin Diseases. A complete Text-Book, with Colored Plates and numerous Wood Engravings. 8vo.
Cloth, 4.50; Leather, 5.50

Van Harlingen on Skin Diseases. A Handbook of the Diseases of the Skin, their Diagnosis and Treatment (arranged alphabetically). By Arthur Van Harlingen, M.D., Clinical Lecturer on Dermatology, Jefferson Medical College; Prof. of Diseases of the Skin in the Philadelphia Polyclinic. 2d Edition. Enlarged. With colored and other plates and illustrations. 12mo. Cloth, 2.50

☞ *See pages 2 to 5 for list of New Manuals.*

SURGERY AND BANDAGING.

Moullin's Surgery, A new Text-Book. 500 Illustrations, 200 of which are original. Cloth, 7.00; Leather, 8.00

Jacobson. Operations in Surgery. A Systematic Handbook for Physicians, Students and Hospital Surgeons. By W. H. A. Jacobson, B.A., Oxon. F.R.C.S. Eng.; Ass't Surgeon Guy's Hospital; Surgeon at Royal Hospital for Children and Women, etc. 199 Illustrations. 1006 pages. 8vo. Cloth. 5.00; Leather, 6.00

Heath's Minor Surgery, and Bandaging. Ninth Edition. 142 Illustrations. 60 Formulæ and Diet Lists. Cloth, 2.00

Horwitz's Compend of Surgery, Minor Surgery and Bandaging, Amputations, Fractures, Dislocations, Surgical Diseases, and the Latest Antiseptic Rules, etc., with Differential Diagnosis and Treatment. By ORVILLE HORWITZ, B.S., M.D., Demonstrator of Surgery, Jefferson Medical College. 4th edition. Enlarged and Rearranged. 136 Illustrations and 84 Formulæ. 12mo. Cloth, 1.00; Interleaved for the addition of Notes, 1.25 *₊* The new Section on Bandaging and Surgical Dressings, consists of 32 Pages and 41 Illustrations. Every Bandage of any importance is figured. This, with the Section on Ligation of Arteries, forms an ample Text-book for the Surgical Laboratory.

Walsham. Manual of Practical Surgery. For Students and Physicians. By WM. J. WALSHAM, M.D., F.R.C.S., Asst. Surg. to, and Dem. of Practical Surg. in, St. Bartholomew's Hospital, Surgeon to Metropolitan Free Hospital, London. With 236 Engravings. *See Page 2.* Cloth, 3.00; Leather, 3.50

URINE, URINARY ORGANS, ETC.

Holland. The Urine, and Common Poisons and The Milk. Chemical and Microscopical, for Laboratory Use. Illustrated. Fourth Edition. 12mo. Interleaved. Cloth, 1.00

Ralfe. Kidney Diseases and Urinary Derangements. 42 Illustrations. 12mo. 572 pages. Cloth, 2.75

Marshall and Smith. On the Urine. The Chemical Analysis of the Urine. By John Marshall, M.D., Chemical Laboratory, Univ. of Penna; and Prof. E. F. Smith, PH.D. Col. Plates. Cloth, 1.00

Tyson. On the Urine. A Practical Guide to the Examination of Urine. With Colored Plates and Wood Engravings. 7th Ed. Enlarged. 12mo. Cloth, 1.50

Van Nüys, Urine Analysis. Illus. Cloth, 2.00

VENEREAL DISEASES.

Hill and Cooper. Student's Manual of Venereal Diseases, with Formulæ. Fourth Edition. 12mo. Cloth, 1.00

☞ *See pages 14 and 15 for list of ! Quiz-Compends !*

BLAKISTON'S ? QUIZ-COMPENDS ?

Bound in Cloth, $1. Interleaved, for the Addition of Notes, $1.25.

☞ *These books are constantly revised to keep up with the latest teachings and discoveries, so that they contain all the new methods and principles. No series of books are so complete in detail, concise in language, or so well printed and bound. Each one forms a complete set of notes upon the subject under consideration.*

Illustrated Descriptive Circular Free.

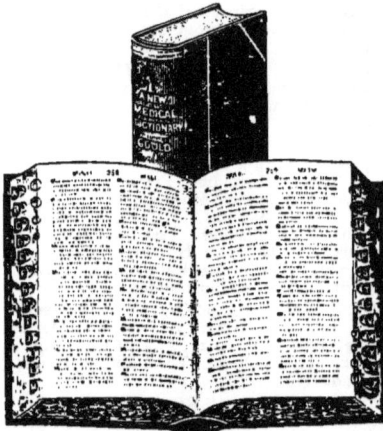

www.ingramcontent.com/pod-product-compliance
Lightning Source LLC
Chambersburg PA
CBHW021509210326
41599CB00012B/1195